D0285278

Foxy
Forever

Also by Noreen Wald

*Contestant: Success Secrets of a
Game Show Veteran*

GHOSTWRITER MYSTERY SERIES:

Death Comes for the Critic

Ghostwriter

Foxy Forever

How to Be Foxy at Fifty,

Sexy at Sixty,

and Fabulous Forever

Noreen Wald

St. Martin's Griffin New York

FOXY FOREVER: HOW TO BE FOXY AT FIFTY, SEXY AT SIXTY, AND FABULOUS FOREVER. Copyright © 2000 by Noreen Wald. All rights reserved. Printed in the United States of America. No part of this book may be used or reproduced in any manner whatsoever without written permission except in the case of brief quotations embodied in critical articles or reviews. For information, address St. Martin's Press, 175 Fifth Avenue, New York, N.Y. 10010.

www.stmartins.com

Book design by Donna Sinsgalli

Library of Congress Cataloging–in–Publication Data

Wald, Noreen.
    Foxy forever : how to be foxy at fifty, sexy at sixty, and fabulous forever / Noreen Wald—1st St. Martin's Griffin ed.
        p. cm.
    ISBN 0-312-25388-5 (pbk.)
    1. Middle-aged women—Life skills guides.   I. Title.

HQ1059.4.W35 2000
646.7'0084'4—dc21

                                                                00-027841

First Edition: June 2000

10   9   8   7   6   5   4   3   2   1

To Doris Holland and Diane Dowling Dufour—

foxy forever and forever friends—

with love

Contents

Acknowledgments

To Every WOW (Wonderful Older Woman)

Thanks for being foxy forever and for sharing your stories with me.

The strengths and struggles, the dreams and disappointments, the loves and losses of each forever WOW who so generously welcomed me into her life have made this book possible: Karen Bartholomew, Vesna Ostertag Beck, Rosalie Bernstein, Helen Brennan, Bernice Crudden, Diane Dowling Dufour, Barbara Giorgio, Martha Gross, Sue Gwinn, Doris Holland, Ellen Johnson, Susan Kavanagh, Agnes Kelly, Barbara Kelly, Betty MacCloskey, Mary Malloy, Joan Mazza, Anne Mulder, Eleanor Nash-Brown, Bonnie Parrish, Gloria Rothstein, and Sandy Young.

And Gloria Stuart and Joyce Sweeney—still too young to be called a WOW but real foxes!

And thanks for the memories of two eternal Wonderful Older Women: Mary Fahy Celeste and Janine Holcombe.

Introduction

Are you about to kiss your forties a none-too-fond farewell? Or are you an early boomer who is—to your amazement—a few years over the half-century mark? Or are you like me, a woman who grew up believing that Father knows best, God or at the very least our husbands would provide, and J. Edgar Hoover was straight?

Not to fret! *Foxy Forever* is both a salute to our past and a prescription for our future. Its game plan is to turn us all into winners, a purposeful, attractive, healthy, amusing, wise, exciting WOW . . . Wonderful Older Woman.

The *Foxy Forever* formula is custom-designed for all women who have ever asked themselves, "What will I be like at fifty . . . sixty . . . seventy? Or ninety? Can there really be a good life after your chin, breasts, and butts have dropped, your gums have receded, your waist has thickened, and your hair has thinned?" The boomers—as well as the generations directly fore and aft of them—will be delighted to know the answers to those questions are: *Awesome* and *Yes!*

I had race-walked with great trepidation toward senior citizenship, looking longingly over my shoulder at my faded youth, resenting impending old age, and suffering from self-doubt and sagging upper arms. After a mini metaphysical moment (see Chapter 1) I became determined to find a formula to help me face and embrace the future. I'd considered myself in relatively good shape mentally, physically, and emotionally; in retrospect, however, I should have started my search sooner. But now I've completed the legwork, and in *Foxy Forever* I share the surprising results.

My path included research. Betty Freidan's *Fountain of Age* proved a somber undertaking; it took two months to wade through and left me feeling sad. In *Late Show*, Helen Gurley Brown sounded so shallow that she made me feel like Mother Teresa. Between the two extremes had to be reality—a workable program for body and soul.

Some of us handle aging with aplomb; many of us face it with fear. I spoke to old friends and dozens of new friends—married, divorced, and single women from fifty to ninety-five. I visited senior citizen groups, doctors, sociologists, cosmetic consultants, hairstylists, a personal trainer, a nutritionist, a past life therapist, and a psychic, thinking things might be better in the world beyond.

Niels Bohr said, "Life can only be understood backward, but it must be lived forward." The past may set us free, but it also has shaped us— literally and figuratively—so I also had to look back at mine before I could move forward. Forevermore may be shorter than before, but as my soul searching revealed, it's still one day at a time. And they can be the best days of our lives.

Foxy Forever provides every Wonderful Older Woman—WOW— with a program to test our limitless potential as we age, aiming for an open mind, a soul with spirit, and a body electric—well, except for my upper arms. Hey, it's progress, not perfection.

And if you don't believe that many women improve with age, check out Hillary Clinton, Jane Pauley, and Leslie Stahl's photos from twenty years ago. The *Foxy Forever* formula challenges us to work on body tissues and soul issues as we accept, embrace, and even enjoy aging.

Foxy at Fifty, Sexy at Sixty, and Fabulous Forever

How to march forward without age getting in our face, our attitude, or our way.

How to be a Goldie Hawn fox in your fifties, Steinemesque in your sixties, and, like Barbara Walters, fascinate your audience forever.

How to star at any dinner party . . . even if you're the extra woman. You're a WOW!

How to accept . . . and admit . . . we're growing old. You have a bunch of famous boomers along for the trip, and they get to celebrate their birthdays in *People* magazine.

A foxy lady both delights and crosses many generations. By becoming a WOW, you can be *Foxy Forever*.

For the
WOW Generation

Foxy forever!

As Time Goes By

"Atrophied vagina" written boldly in the space provided for diagnosis on the health insurance form certainly caught my attention. For God's sake, hadn't the doctor told me not fifteen minutes before, with my feet up in stirrups and the Pap smear completed, "You're in great shape for the shape you're in"?

An atrophied vagina—I'd always figured that would be a near death experience! How had this happened? I looked pretty good on the outside. Well, a little looser in the jaw and a lot lower in the buttocks, but I still turned a few heads, if arthritis hadn't made their necks too stiff to swivel, and I still wore a size 6. Would tearing up the insurance form, paying in cash, and swearing the receptionist to secrecy cover the paper trail? Or would it be better to hire a hit man to give the gynecologist an internal he'd never forget?

Age is a sneak. There I'd been moussed, tinted, toned—well, that's a stretch—cholesterol free, calcium filled, swabbing selected body parts with sunscreen lotion ranging from 4 to 45, sort of an adult's paint-by-the-numbers game. How could my insides have had the audacity to shrivel?

While I was busy running in the other direction, age seemed not only to have caught up but to have delivered a cruel blow beneath the belt, so to speak. Despite my best efforts to the contrary, I'd arrived at a place in life I never expected to be: postmenopausal and pre–Social Security. And like many of us, I'd given it little thought and less planning. Yesterday, or so it seems, I partied, twisting the night away in my mini. Invitations had kept coming: I've had entree to AARP for years, Senior Partners Banking, which doesn't save you a penny (though I have enjoyed the lower senior prices at many movie theaters), and discounted rides at Disney World. God only knew what thrills tomorrow would bring.

Up to then I had managed to ignore both the invitations and the calendar. I even moved to Florida, the only place in the world where you can be an ingenue at fifty. Really old people scared me, so I had avoided them, too, which is not easy in Pompano Beach where ubiquitous mortality, dressed in Easter-egg-pastel polyester pantsuits with elastic waists confronted you daily.

Ironically, I'd chosen to revel in the past, far preferring nostalgia and old movies to reality while living a script that didn't have a last act. And why not? It was a great role; I enjoyed playing the part. Not serendipity, but even sans husband or a high-powered career life was good. Often damn good.

I'd reached an age that gave me automatic acceptance in some retirement homes, yet I worked harder at physical well-being than ever before, doing aerobics in the pool most mornings. I was much more grateful for manageable hair and a slim frame than I'd been at thirty. Both were accidents of genes rather than design. Yet despite decades of working in the fashion and beauty industries, I would occasionally buy a beautifully packaged ninety-five-dollar jar of grease that promised to stave off the ravages of time. I applied makeup with the deft touch achieved by eons of practice and plucked gray hairs from my brow with the skill of a surgeon. If I didn't slow down the plucking, I'd have alopecia of the eyebrows. But when the lights over the mirror were pink enough and with eyeglasses vision that was less than acute, it had seemed worth the effort. I'd requested that my cosmetic bag and my rosary beads be tucked into my casket for the same reason, just in case.

Control has always been an issue—big time. I've always preferred being in charge. And I had believed I had the solution to most of life's problems, figuring that if you kept the outside wrappings tight and shiny, the package wouldn't unravel. However, that day in the doctor's office, as I faced the receptionist and the diagnosis, my usual optimistic attitude was seriously challenged. No matter how much I resented it or rouged the other cheek, I was getting older, and it was out of my control. Scary. Would I wind up being afraid of me?

When my periods had started playing hide and seek, here one month, missing the next two or three, I decided not to go on estrogen, alone or paired with progesterone. The history of cancer in my family was paramount in my decision. A woman gynecologist in Manhattan had concurred.

Would this be my reward for having chosen—possibly for the first time in my life—health over vanity? I knew that once my estrogen took a hike, osteoporosis might or might not arrive, my sex drive might or might not diminish, and I might or might not have ghastly night sweats, nervous fits, or the vapors. I'd gone the calcium and exercise route, trusting my bones would hold me up straight. And so far none of the above had plagued me. Did this grim prognosis bode a worse diagnosis?

A blurb in *Vogue* magazine later revealed the surprising results of a Clinique Truth/Beauty Survey, a nationwide poll that attempted to discover how women really felt about getting older. Notice that wording—not growing old, not aging, but the sugar-coated "getting older." Most of the women polled had considered fifty-four "the end of youth." On the day of the infamous diagnosis I'd already passed that milestone. Never mind ruing the end of youth; what I felt qualified as panic.

And I just kept "getting older"! I'd considered myself a fighter and a survivor; however, it's easy to be spunky when you believe the problem you're facing will have a positive resolution. Growing old seemed totally negative, and facing old age cheerfully an oxymoron. While I had no plans to go gently into that final good night, aging proved more than tough to accept: It was goddamn depressing. If depression is anger turned inward—Group Therapy 101—I'd better do a pirouette and segue into an attitude adjustment. Ready or not, Act 3 would be coming up. I knew I wanted writer's credit!

After that dreadful day at the doctor's I remember driving home on a road parallel to the ocean, parking the car, taking off my shoes, and hitting the beach. The sea comforts me. A true Cancer the crab, a water sign.

I love the beach in real life and in the movies. Deborah Kerr and a young Burt Lancaster locked in sand-covered sex as the waves rolled in; Holly Hunter with her piano in a sand trap, only to be rescued by a surprisingly sexy Harvey Keitel; *Beaches*, the sandy beginning and ending for Bette Midler and Barbara Hershey; a young Susan Sarandon and an old Burt Lancaster on the boardwalk in *Atlantic City*. I have great faith that somewhere on a beach in eternity I'll run into Burt.

It had been raining just before I left the car. As Floridians say, "If you don't like the weather, wait five minutes." As if drawn with a brush stroke, a rainbow appeared. Its colors turned the sultry late-afternoon sky into a glorious picture. Did the Pleiades have a day job painting rainbows? The sky brightened, and so did my mood. Breathing the ocean air, I had a mini awakening, a low-grade spiritual experience. Take this age thing a day at a time. Carpe diem. An atrophied vagina isn't fatal. It turned out to be less than an inconvenience. Romance and Replens (an over-the-counter lubricant) can conquer all.

A later reevaluation of estrogen therapy with my current doctor changed my mind and my body! With a daily dose of Prempro, the problem is history.

The time had come to accept and admit that I would grow old. No matter how clever we are, there's no way to beat the clock—and I certainly wanted it to keep on ticking. Though I didn't know it then, I'd stumbled on the first step to becoming a WOW. Over the next several years I searched for and found an irreverent, pragmatic, healthy, and, yes, fun formula for growing old . . . while remaining foxy forever.

I knew I had to begin major work on my resentment of aging. Though I'll never wear polyester pantsuits and I'll always believe Easter-egg pastels look better in nurseries—some chic babies, if asked, might prefer checks or plaids—I decided that my acceptance of the aging process would be essential to my happiness. My attitude, along with my body and soul, had to change.

I also knew change is a bitch.

Sentimental Journey

The Way We Were is how we got to be the way we are. Wedged between the two most famous generations in America's history, mine is a generation with no name. Rona Jaffe called us the Do-Nothing Generation, but she's wrong. We did do something. We went to the movies.

My yesterdays were spent at double features complete with serial, Warner's Pathé-News, a Bugs Bunny cartoon, a contraband bag of White Castle hamburgers, and an orange crush. Fifty years later I still can't watch *Double Indemnity* or the original *The Postman Always Rings Twice* without smelling those onions and pickles.

The war and I hit the movies at about the same time. My grandmother Etta had a thing for Errol Flynn. The Colony, a neighborhood rerun theater, was screening an Olivia de Havilland and Errol Flynn double bill. Etta brought me along. Lots of swords, tights, teeth, blood, and bodies. I was hooked for life.

In those days, thank God, no one questioned whether a movie could affect a child for good or bad. I saw everything from *Pinocchio* to *Gilda*. I watched Mary Astor go from *The Maltese Falcon*'s smoldering Brigid O'Shaugnessy to *Little Women*'s Marmee in eight short years.

Mostly, however, I went to war: *Bataan, The Purple Heart, Guadalcanal Diary, Thirty Seconds Over Tokyo*. To this day I've never owned a Japanese car.

Bleak and frightening newsreels, together with grim documentaries like *The Battle of the Beaches* and *The Life and Death of the U.S.S. Hornet*, were my early history lessons. Young soldiers were dying on faraway bat-tlefields; children were dying in concentration camps. Who would save the world?

The white hats appeared in the newsreels—Franklin Roosevelt, Winston Churchill, the British royal family. I wanted to grow up and drive an ambulance like Princess Elizabeth. Hitler, Mussolini, and Tojo were evil incarnate, villains straight from central casting.

Everyone did his part. Fonda, Power, Gable, and Stewart enlisted, leaving Van Johnson in Hollywood to fight the battles on the silver screen. Bing Crosby and Bob Hope went on the road to entertain the troops. Ann Sheridan, Betty Grable, and Veronica Lake urged us to buy war bonds at newsreel-covered rallies, and my mom sold saving bonds in the lobby of the Boulevard Theater.

With four hours of pure escapism every Saturday and Sunday, I was programmed to deny reality. My heroines were Jennifer Jones's Bernadette and Greer Garson's Mrs. Miniver. A budding anglophile, I wanted to be a wife and mother who tended roses and rescued German pilots with equal aplomb. My new favorite song was "The White Cliffs of Dover."

Summer Sundays were spent at the beach—Rockaway, where the Atlantic Ocean meets Queens. The "Irish Riviera" consisted of tiny bungalows filled with large families, saloons filled with serious pale drinkers who never made it to the beach, and Playland, an amusement park filled with suntanned kids.

Even here I played movies. Dog-paddling through the waves, I would keep an eye out for U-boats, checking for a periscope of a German submarine. If a young man swam ashore and did not plop on a crowded blanket, I would follow him, certain he was a spy. If he went farther than the boardwalk, democracy was doomed since I wasn't allowed to leave the sand.

I loved to sit and stare across the ocean, wishing I could be Margaret O'Brien, starring as a teary British war orphan in *Journey for Margaret*, or brave Bonita Granville in *Hitler's Children*, defying SS brutality. In retrospect, the latter was rather racy. All those black boots and whips, combined with young buxom blondes flogged for refusing to cohabit with the Nazis.

My day at the beach would end in Bessie the Buick for the ride back to Jackson Heights. Daddy wanted to listen to the Dodgers; I wanted to listen to "The Shadow." Red Barber's calls filled the car far more often than "Who knows what evil lurks in the hearts of men?"

When not watching the war on screen, we played war in the streets. A big chalk globe was sectioned into six or seven wedges. Each kid stood in a wedge that represented a country. We chose our countries from the newsreels—Czechoslovakia, Poland, Hungry, Turkey, Russia, China. One kid stood in the center of the circle and bounced a Spalding into a wedge shouting, "I declare war on Turkey!" or whichever country caught his little Fascist fancy. Alliances were formed, and a series of Spalding maneuvers decided the victors.

We played movies indoors as well. Dressed in my mother's girlfriend's discarded white halter and with my hair wrapped in a white towel-turban, I *was* Lana Turner. Then we had Betty Grable, Rita Hayworth, and Lana paper dolls, complete with cutout costumes from their hit films. We would play for hours with dialogue taken directly from sappy quotes in *Photoplay* or *Modern Screen*. By nine, wearing my mother's cartwheel hat, I was a regular Hedda Hopper.

On V-J Day, I was at Times Square surrounded by a sea of white sailor suits and a field of Army and Marine hats jaunty above fresh young faces. The crowd was patriotic pandemonium.

In my starched pinafore braided blond hair, scrubbed and shining outside, bursting with pride and confidence in God's country inside, a child of the forties, I knew this would make a great movie.

The identification with strong women continued with Myrna Loy's quintessential postwar wife and mother in 1946's *The Best Years of Our Lives*. A less traditional mother was played by Robin Hood's old girlfriend, Olivia de Havilland, in *To Each His Own*. My mother had taken me to see this "woman's" picture, and she immediately regretted it. I remember asking loudly, "Mom, how could she have a baby when she isn't married?" This led to an abridged mother-daughter sex talk. In our Irish-Catholic home, sex, like the Holy Trinity, remained a mystery.

In the late forties, with propaganda movies no longer relevant, Hollywood turned to social issues. The medium was the message, and often it was right on target. *Lost Weekend* presented alcoholism as an ugly disease, with Ray Milland's forlorn drunk as its victim. Gregory Peck's Phil Green in *Gentleman's Agreement*, proved anti-Semitism hadn't died with Germany's defeat; it was here in America, hiding in the closets of restricted hotels and the locker rooms of country clubs. *Johnny Belinda* covered the rape of a deaf mute. The heroine kept her illegitimate baby, a stigma in 1948. Jane Wyman—Ronald Reagan's first wife—won an Oscar for her role as Belinda. *To Each His Own* had taught me that an unmarried woman can have a baby. *Johnny Belinda* taught me that love can win over adversity. Two valuable lessons.

The decade ended, and so did my childhood. I was off to Manhattan, enrolled in the Dominican Academy, a Catholic preparatory school for young ladies. Miscast again!

Audrey Hepburn's princess from an unnamed country, in *Roman Holiday*, had me rolling up the sleeves on my white uniform blouse, adding a wide belt to my New Look full skirt, and cutting off my shoulder-length mane to achieve Hepburn's pixie hairstyle. It looked a hell of a lot better on her! I tried to walk and talk in her ladylike manner, too, and even began to pay attention to my ballet and etiquette classes. The nuns were puzzled but pleased. It was 1953, and most teenage girls wanted to be Audrey. Or Liz.

A Place in the Sun was the sexiest movie I had ever seen. Elizabeth Taylor was so lush, Montgomery Clift so gorgeous, and Shelley Winters so expendable—I would have drowned her on their behalf. Liz's strapless ball gown became the dream prom dress of the decade. Or Marilyn. Monroe's Lorelei Lee in *Gentlemen Prefer Blondes* drove lots of us to the Light and Bright bottle. I learned all the words to "Diamonds Are a Girl's Best Friend" and would sing them in an off-key but passable imitation of Marilyn's whispery tones. The padded push-up bras proved less successful.

And then along came Grace.

Mogambo pitted Kelly against Ava Gardner for Gable, who was reprising his big white hunter role from *Red Dust* twenty-one years earlier. In that version Mary Astor had challenged Jean Harlow for his affections.

Jean was long dead, Mary was long relegated to mother roles, but King Clark, a quarter of a century older than his current leading ladies, was still roaring for MGM. Any pity for Mary's plight vanished as Grace in designer safari attire—*Out of Africa* meets Ralph Lauren—appeared on the screen.

To Catch a Thief starred Grace, Cary Grant, and the French Riviera. It's hard to say which of the three was the most beautiful. This was Hitchcock at his classiest. Jessie Royce Landis, who was so wonderful as stuffy Grace's down-to-earth mom, was younger than Kelly's suitor, Cary Grant. My generation bought into the message: Men age so well that they can court their contemporaries' daughters. Older women get to play mothers.

I was desperate to be an Alfred Hitchcock heroine: cool, blond, slim, smart, and often with a job. In *Rear Window*, Grace Kelly worked for a magazine and dressed like a *Vogue* model. Eva Marie Saint in *North by Northwest* was a double agent. Even Kim Novak in the convoluted *Vertigo* held a job, at least in one of her two identities. But not being as cool, blond, or smart as a Hitchcock heroine, I married the first man who asked me.

By the mid-fifties, Grace and I were both planning church weddings. She was an Oscar-winning, twenty-seven-year-old movie star marrying a reigning European monarch. I was a college student, almost nineteen, marrying a neighborhood ex-Marine. Both grooms looked dashing in their respective uniforms.

The *Journal-American's* Cholly Knickerbocker column had replaced *Photoplay* and *Modern Screen* as my chief source of entertainment news. I followed Grace's wedding with far more interest than my own. The cost of her wedding gown exceeded my ex-Marine's annual wage. Mine didn't. My father joked that we should just let down the hem on my first communion dress. The family was less than happy that I would be marrying two years before I could vote. However, with my mother's credit card in hand, I headed for Lord & Taylor. My dress was worthy of a movie bride, with me cast as a cross between Audrey's and Grace's princess roles. Unfortunately, in the wedding pictures I looked more like Sandra Dee, minus the eye makeup.

In 1961, Audrey Hepburn, starring as *Breakfast at Tiffany's* Holly

Golightly, was reinstated as my forever-favorite movie star. Holly's little black sleeveless dress—actually an off-the-rack copy—and her big black sunglasses became my fashion staples for decades. How I wished I could have attended one of Holly's parties! Instead I was very married and about to become a mother. I did take to hanging out in Tiffany's on a regular basis, never buying anything except at their January Christmas card sale; like Holly, I found it a comforting place.

Suddenly stealing the scenes from all the movie stars was JACKIE!

Hollywood stars were our royalty. Now the venue had switched to Washington. Jacqueline Bouvier Kennedy was married to our thirty-fifth president, John Fitzgerald Kennedy, scion of an Irish-American family with lacier curtains than mine. Their son, John-John, was born in November 1960. Our son, Billy, in May 1961. Just as I tried to become Jackie's mirror image—poofed hair and narrow silhouettes—Billy became John-John's clone, with long bangs and Eton collars.

The country and I couldn't get enough of Jackie. Our love affair with Camelot's heroine lasted over thirty years.

I devoured game shows as an intellectual break from changing diapers and preparing formula. My first appearance as a contestant, resulting from my mother's cajoling, was on *Password*'s evening show in the spring of '62.

My costars were Jane Fonda and James Mason. That year Henry's daughter, Jane, was a Broadway ingenue. James Mason, long a major motion picture star both in Britain and the U.S.A. played an elegant villain. His eloquent voice was orgasmic. I found myself sandwiched between the two of them.

My opening night on *Password* resulted in a *TV Guide* photo spread with Jane and James. I thought I'd climbed a real-life *Stairway to Heaven*. That show was the first of seven contestant stints—yes, including *Jeopardy!*—where Movies and Religion were the good categories and World History the nemesis. My first book, *Contestant*, published in the middle of my search for *Foxy Forever*'s formula, reveals my secrets as a game show veteran and is also a step-by-step guide—a how-to—for the reader to get on a show, play, and win.

Part-time work on pilot TV shows for Goodson-Todman and Merv Griffin Productions followed my appearances on *Password* and *Jeopardy!* I was being paid to play games with the stars. Fantasy merged with reality. My husband might become as expendable as Shelley Winters.

Both my parents died within a year. After their house was sold, while I was still grieving, we moved to the suburbs. The movies, as always, offered escape and solace, though they were now located in a mall, a poor substitute for the gilded and velvet movie palaces of my youth.

Identification was trickier. Doris Day's forty-plus virgins romped through several hits saying no to Rock Hudson. Lana Turner was now *Madame X*, complete with rigid hair and emotional range. Anne Bancroft's bored Mrs. Robinson was a scary harbinger of what happened to marriages of a certain age.

Movie censorship was out. A rating system replaced the long-running Hays Code. Sex and violence became main attractions. Change was in.

Faye Dunaway's depression chic in *Bonnie and Clyde*, as she shot up middle America, and Mia Farrow's boyish haircut in *Rosemary's Baby*, as she had sex with the devil, became fashion statements. For the first time in my life some of Hollywood's leading ladies were younger than I, and glamour, as I knew it, was gone from the silver screen.

In the seventies, *The Turning Point* and *Julia* focused on women's friendships. In the former, frustrated ballerina Shirley MacLaine and Anne Bancroft, as a prima past her prime, had a fistfight to remember. Jane Fonda's Lillian Hellman thwarted the Nazis with a push from Vanessa Redgrave's *Julia*. Jane had come a long way from our *Password* game. I had come a long way, too.

Jill Clayburgh starred as *An Unmarried Woman* in 1978, but I held the title a year before she did. Neither the man I'd divorced nor the ones I eventually dated seemed as interesting as Clayburgh's former and future loves. I blamed this sad state of affairs on New Jersey, and moved to Manhattan, the land of opportunity for Jill's character. I had a new job and a new apartment, and my own Blue Cross/Blue Shield. I started wearing Jill's unmarried woman's sleepwear—cotton T-shirt and underpants. Still do. But I never did meet anyone as intriguing as the men in that movie.

My son was a college freshman. His mother was playing a Katharine Hepburn career gal, on location in the Chrysler Building, with a secretary who had never heard of Rita Hayworth. My New York City role in the early eighties was a far cry from *Woman of the Year*. The unkindest cut was a work scene so busy, I couldn't get my cinematic fix.

A VCR and the AMC channel brought the movies home. I could watch at any hour in any garb. DeMille, Spielberg, Wilder, and Hitchcock spike my cornflakes and bananas with genius.

Down, depressed, or just dog-tired, I could replay Dooley Wilson singing "As Time Goes By" for Ingrid Bergman's Ilsa or Paul Henreid lighting two cigarettes as Bette Davis settled for the stars in *Now, Voyager*. Or *Mr. Skeffington*, where Bette was her usual bitchy self and Claude Rains her long-suffering husband. Bette grew old and scarred, and Claude's character went blind, remembering her only as the beautiful young woman he had married. Hollywood's convenient answer to aging.

When I first watched Bette Davis star in those movies, she was more than twenty-five years older than I. In her close-ups, filling my small screen, she would always be much younger.

On my more recent—though less frequent—trips to the movies, I've observed a return to the Cinderella story. *Pretty Woman*'s plot turned a hooker with a heart of gold and big teeth into a millionaire's wife. Staten Island's *Working Girl* wound up with both her snooty upper-class boss's career and her boyfriend. Jane Austen, the Brontës, and Shakespeare have once again become big box office.

And as time goes by I realize that despite decades of chasing after glamour and grande dame roles, I've remained emotionally more like Gidget than either Mrs. Miniver or Mrs. Robinson.

Ac-cen-chu-ate
the Positive

Some reflection seemed in order. Why was I what I was? A woman of a certain age who found herself wistfully humming "Someone to Watch Over Me" while loudly proclaiming that she was single by choice, was self-supporting, cherished her independence, and would never share a bathroom. *What was going on?*

An identity crisis can pop up at any stage of life, but it became a serious nuisance when I was running out of time to find myself.

The solitary journey, which had seemed the only way to go for so many years, sometimes loomed lonely. An intense urge to find a partner, a primal mating call, would revisit, and then just as suddenly vanish. Ambivalence had become constant.

And not only in affairs—or the lack of affairs—of the heart. A fizzled romance had been one of the reasons I'd escaped from Manhattan. Here I stood, kicking sand on the shore, when I wanted to pound the pavement on Madison Avenue. Could I have both? Should I return to my roots? Should I move to a whaling village? Sag Harbor sounded good.

I flew to New York, drove to the Hamptons, checked it out, and returned undecided. Indecision ran rampant, which was tough for a gal who ranked impulsiveness just above godliness. Cleanliness, as adaged, came next in the pecking order.

A noisy committee, holding a myriad of opinions and questions, chaired the meeting in my mind. What did I want? Why was I living so far away from my family? Who did I need in my life, if anyone? Was growing old the problem? The answer to the last question looked like a definite maybe.

Katharine Hepburn had once told Dick Cavett that she found no redeeming factor in growing old. If Kate, a legend and one of my heroines, had felt that way, how would mere mortals fare? Could Kate have been wrong? Could my attitude suck?

In an attempt to adjust to the inevitable while attempting to restore and keep my usual ebullience intact, I headed to the library. Like Francie Nolan in *A Tree Grows in Brooklyn*, I'd always wanted to start with the A's and read through the alphabet. Fiction. I'd avoided self-help books like the plague. Maybe I would reconsider my options and check them out.

Both Betty Freidan and Helen Gurley Brown had written books on aging. Betty's *Fountain of Age* solved the paucity in the men-to-women ratio by suggesting that two old gals could share one old guy. In *Late Show*, this was Helen's cosmopolitan advice: "If I were alone and sexually needy and no single man was available [likely], I would borrow a husband—preferably of a wife I didn't know—just as I did when I was single and younger." I don't think so, Helen.

I couldn't travel either of those paths. I'd stumbled on the first step toward change, but I hadn't climbed any higher. I knew I would have to find my own formula for successful aging. And I'd better get moving. Growing old was no longer around the corner; I was standing in the vestibule.

During the summer of '95, Helen Gurley Brown spurred me on. The war in Bosnia had escalated into NATO air strikes. O. J. Simpson's trial held the country rapt. Chicago's heat wave had resulted in five hundred dead, and counting. The Senate was investigating Whitewater, Waco, and Packwood, while Helen was busy choosing *Cosmopolitan*'s first male centerfold since Burt Reynolds in the early seventies. CNN presented Helen in a pink, puff-sleeved baby doll dress, too many inches above her knees, wearing a wig atop her too tight face. Two of the contestants hoisted her

1. *Admit* and accept that you are no longer young. Your audience already knows it!
2. *Believe* that your personal best is yet to come.
3. *Create* an ageless attitude; turn it into an ageless lifestyle.
4. *Perform* at Oscar-winning capacity. Act 3 is your pièce de résistance.
5. *Enjoy* yourself. Eliminate negativity. No one—except maybe your best friend—wants to hear it.
6. *Allow* new ideas, new people, and new goals to enter your life.
7. *Keep* changing. Happiness is change. To hold on to it, you have to give it away.

above their heads—not too difficult a feat since Helen was a paper-thin slip of a seventy-plus cosmopolitan girl.

Never had I been more grateful to Katharine Hepburn and Marlene Dietrich for turning well-cut trousers and simple tailored shirts into a classic woman's ageless look.

I soul-searched all summer. And researched. And talked to other women. Single. Long-married. Divorced. Remarried. Widowed. Seniors. Boomers. Rich. Poor. Religious. Atheists. Sexually active. Celibates. Working. Retired. Optimists. Pessimists.

I learned from these women—those who shared my fears and those who had successfully conquered their fears.

Reflection led to change. Change led to action. Action led to *Foxy Forever*'s seven-step formula. Following that formula, I changed not only my attitude but my career, my city, and my life. Its steps, offering the antidote to fear of aging, are both a paean to our past and a prescription for our future. An R_x for a happy, healthy old age . . . living each day as a WOW!

ABC + PEAK = FOXY FOREVER!

"Yeah, yeah," you may say. "Easier written than lived." This is true, but take a closer look at the seven steps and see how each of them can work for you if you work them.

Admit and accept that you are no longer young. Your audience already knows it.   If you're a boomer, you're still hanging out in the vestibule, but you'd better be prepared when that door swings open. Senior citizenship is lurking there, waiting for you. But you need not fear. Your slightly older sisters—we women in the vanguard who are about to become the first young/old generation—will be there to greet you.

As women who grew up believing father knew best, we were too busy polishing our Danish modern furniture and toilet-training toddlers to burn our bras. We were a generation at first confused and then later provoked into small changes by the women's movement.

Women who came of age in the fifties enjoyed being girls. Lacy garter belts held up our seamed hose. Lacy padded bras held up our bosoms, permitting the teeniest amount of ladylike cleavage to show. We wore waist cinchers under our wide belts and multiple lacy crinolines under our full circle skirts. I had to turn sideways to negotiate a subway door. We often added a panty girdle under all those layers, but Superman's X-ray vision couldn't have found our tummies or our butts. We looked more like lampshades than hourglasses.

Clean was cool. Well groomed was de rigueur. The scarlet polish on our fingernails matched the polish on our toes. Grunge would never have made it as a fashion statement in 1959.

We dressed for men, either to attract one or to keep one. I know that's a shameful secret, long locked in the closet, but listen, over forty years have gone by, we can finally fess up.

The thing was, it worked. Our audience was responsive; they, too, enjoyed watching us being girls.

It worked for decades. I remember on a trip to Mexico, circa 1971, catching a full-length view of myself in a hotel mirror and thinking how idiotic I looked—heading out for dinner in hot pants . . . because they were in style!

But did I change? No way. Not my pants or my attitude. Well into my thirties, I still enjoyed being a girl.

Two decades later I knew that my audience had waned. Oh, a handful would still applaud a new and, by that time, far more age-appropriate outfit or hairdo, but center stage was held by much younger players.

I had admitted I was no longer young; now I had to accept it.

Guess what. With acceptance came freedom. Gone was bondage to unflattering fads, tortured hairdos, and tight underwear. Acceptance meant that who I am matters more than what I look like.

Well, most of the time.

Believe that your personal best is yet to come. If we think it's all over, it probably is. If we believe that our best years are history, they will be.

Angela Lansbury became younger as she grew older. When she played Laurence Harvey's wicked mother in *The Manchurian Candidate*, she was a year younger than he. Lansbury told Larry King, "As an actress, age doesn't have any bearing on the ability to look forward with joy. It simply opens up new pages of possibilities." Substitute "woman" for "actress," and you have the second step.

New Passages author Gail Sheehy believes postmenopausal women often get a new energy along with a second childhood. A second wind. That has been true for me. Lazy by nature (just ask my ex-husband), I prefer lounging in bed reading to doing almost anything else—especially working out. Yet I'm anti-osteoporosis and pro-exercise to prevent it.

Poor posture can be a real monkey on your back: a dowager's hump. Proper vertebrae stretches will allow you to stand tall and straight—two good reasons to get me moving. Now I try to arrange my schedule around a four-day-a-week workout: aerobics and stretches as well as walking. Not too tough. After all, it is only an elevator ride from my apartment down to the gym. Reluctantly crawling out of bed or away from my writing, I emerge from my exercise feeling better psychologically, philosophically, and physiologically.

I'll never race-walk the ten-minute mile; I never did. Yet I feel great and look good, and my blood pressure is 110/60.

Set personal goals—always achievable. As you see results, you will want to increase the objectives. Come to believe:

- A bad habit takes six weeks to break.
- A love affair takes six weeks to get over.
- An exercise program takes six weeks to become a habit.
- A habit takes six weeks to turn into a love affair.

Personal best should include clever makeup, a great haircut, and classic clothes. Our fifties, sixties, seventies, and beyond can be the foxiest days of our lives. "The last of life for which the first was made." Thank you, Robert Burns.

Create an ageless attitude; turn it into an ageless lifestyle. A woman of a certain age can now rest assured that that term covers a long time span and has become unisex. Wonderful news for those of us who have been a certain age for ages!

William Safire's "On Language" column in the Sunday *New York Times Magazine* once posed the question, "How old is a woman of a certain age?" His answer: "Only a Nosy Parker would try to find out. But the expression is becoming androgynous, and the age seems to be creeping upward."

Ageless, when spoken as a compliment, seldom refers to appearance but rather to an attitude, a *je ne sais quoi*, transcending body and soul, and encouraging others to bask in its glow. The quality that allows Generation X and Tom Brokaw's Greatest Generation—our elders—to become equally intrigued in our presence. An ability to entertain and to be entertained by the company we're currently keeping.

If the crowd is twenty-something, the conversation isn't likely to include "What a damn shame the folks born in 1917 are being screwed by the Social Security system." However, when chatting with the World War II generation, it's a hot topic.

And the AMC channel has shown many members of Generation X that Cameron Diaz is no Grace Kelly. So we don't need to point that out.

Eclectic decorators are in demand, and so are eclectic communicators. An interior designer who offers a roomful of various periods and styles is sure to please some passers-through. An ageless attitude will do the same for the lucky people who pass through your life.

A graceful carriage, attractive appearance, and alert mind all help. But it's a genuine interest in others, combined with flexibility, that results in an ageless lifestyle. Not only will we fit into diverse social groups, but we will be sought after and warmly welcomed.

It does take homework. We need to turn off Oprah, pick up a biography of Bernard Baruch, and read it with the Spice Girls singing in the background. That may be going too far. I confess that when Kurt Cobain committed suicide, I never knew he'd ever been alive. Pop music, like nuclear physics, has remained a weak area in my *Jeopardy!* board of life.

Perform at Oscar-winning capacity. Act 3 is your *pièce de résistance.* We Wonderful Older Women get to play the role to the hilt. But best of all, we get to write and direct the script. With the wit and wisdom we've acquired over the decades while we rehearsed or missed cues and responded to the wrong lines, we can now earn rave reviews.

If the program has been bland so far, we can delight our audience with a tart Act 3. If the scenery has gotten stale, we can stage the finale in a new setting. If the plot needs a romantic twist, we can pencil in a love interest. If it doesn't work out, we can erase him. If old grudges need resolution, we can script our amends before the house lights dim. If miserable people with terminal negativity are cluttering front and center stage, like all the dead bodies in the last act of *Hamlet*, we can write them out. We deserve a happy ending. *Foxy Forever* will show the way there.

Enjoy yourself. Eliminate negativity. No one—except maybe your best friend—wants to hear it. I come from a family whose members respond with a full medical report when asked, "How do you feel?" I've watched a glaze come over my listener's eyes and a face blanch in horror—even a doctor's or a nurse's—as I vividly described my acute cystitis. So I learned early on that the response to that question to any nonfamily member should be "Fine, thank you."

That same response should cover questions regarding our souls as well as our bodies. Very few friends and *no* acquaintances want to hear that we feel sad, fat, or unloved. One WOW friend has answered "How are you?" with a cheerful litany: "Jobless, manless, chinless, sexless, and doing great." Her listeners always laughed, knowing that right around the corner she'd have a new job, a good man, a firm chin, and great sex. And that's just what happened. This WOW combined a positive attitude with a witty retort during a time of adversity. We can all do just such an attitude adjustment on a daily or minute-to-minute basis if need be.

Our finest assets are a few good friends—those we can share anything with, who will not only listen but will offer advice and consent when needed, and compassion always. A treasured confidante will see us through a bad time and will love us for ourselves—hypochondria and all. And remember, it's a reciprocal deal.

The world is full of woe, so keep kvetching to a minimum. Don't pollute our social environment with negative remarks, jaded sarcasm, or chronic ennui. If depression seems clinical, see a doctor immediately. Otherwise, volunteer at a hospital, teach a child to read, feed the homeless, or simply listen to someone else's troubles. Yours often will pale by comparison.

Be generous with compliments. Be stingy with any criticism. If a social life is to be included on our agenda—hidden or otherwise—we should schedule "Smile" in our Daytimers as a permanent to-do.

Allow new ideas, new people, and new goals to enter your life. Here are five phrases that guarantee we will be narrow-minded old broads living in a narrow world:

> I always did it this way.
> In my day . . .
> Good manners have vanished.

We had our babies at the traditional age in the traditional manner—
   anesthetized.
No one writes good books anymore.
I don't understand young people these days.

Try:

That's a great idea, I never thought of doing it that way.
We've come so far since I was young.
Please tell me, how can I help you?
That videotape of his birth will certainly impress Danny's first date.
Wasn't Grisham's first book his best? Reminded me of my old favorite,
   To Kill a Mockingbird (a sneaky way to introduce a fledging reader
   to Harper Lee).
What do you think?

My friends' children have become my friends. They choose to have
tea with me when I return to Manhattan. They come to dinner at Mom's
when I'm a house guest there. They even solicit my advice long distance.
My niece and my great-niece are also frequent tea table pals. Best of all,
my son and I love and respect each other. Sometimes he'll even have a
cup of Lipton's with me!

**Keep changing. Happiness is change. To hold on to it,
you have to give it away.**   For decades I believed that happiness
came from having the right man open the right door—the passenger side
of a Mercedes and the hatch of a fifty-foot sloop. This dreamboat would
wear chinos, Docksiders, and a white broadcloth shirt with no logo. He
would own a traditional tux, and he'd dress for dinner. His grammar would
be impeccable, he'd quote Thoreau, and he'd laugh at my jokes. Needless
to say, he has remained a missing person.

   People, places, or things can't make us happy. It's our full-time job
and worth every minute. If we don't change and grow every day, we
stagnate. We won't become perfect—God forbid. Who'd want to be?

However, we will come to know, to accept, and to love ourselves. The real us, complete with aging bodies but forever young souls.

By working the seven steps we can find joy in Act 3. Then we get to give it away. It's returned in a baby's smile, a summer sunset, a finished chapter, or an impulsive kiss. Life happens where we are, not where we were. The days do grow short when we reach September, but we can turn autumn into our prime time!

For the Body

Call me a frivolous fox! Maybe

working on our outside appear-

ance isn't putting first things first,

but looking good can lead to

feeling good!

Put On a Happy Face

What do Audrey Hepburn's Carmelite in *The Nun's Story*, Ellen Burstyn's Jewish widow in *The Cemetery Club*, and Frank Langella's vampire in *Dracula* have in common? Not looking in mirrors.

The Carmelite's convent is devoid of mirrors. The widow's mirrors are all covered while she sits shiva. The vampire has a mirror—wouldn't want guests to get suspicious—but he never sneaks a peek. No image, you understand.

A world without mirrors might be a better place. The ones in movie theaters, flooding our faces with fluorescent lighting, turning our teeth yellow and our laugh lines into furrows, should be X-rated. Use at your own risk.

After sufficient reflection I've decided that powdering my nose in rest rooms located in airports, diners, and most office buildings is masochistic behavior. Wash your hands with your eyes closed or face the fright of your life.

However, any woman who doesn't look good in her own bathroom, bedroom, or living room mirror should change her lightbulbs immediately! Pink side lighting is guaranteed to take off ten years and add a warm glow to our complexions. The hell with looking at the world through rose-colored glasses. I want the world to see me in a rosy glow, at least in my own home. And I want to take that glow on the road. Looking good doesn't happen by accident but by disciplined design.

Some women are sexy at sixty with a dash of lipstick and a splash of eau de cologne. That's a gift from the gods, like an A in geometry or being able to digest cucumbers. Minus makeup, I wasn't even sexy at thirty.

A long-ago move from my New York homestead to my ten-year expatriation in New Jersey involved the installation of three telephones in a brand-new Wedgwood blue colonial. Two installers arrived at eight o'clock on a cold February morning. I greeted them in an old chenille robe, fuzzy slippers, the Wild Woman from Borneo's hairdo, and a naked face. We spent about an hour together, selecting colors and respective locations. This was, of course, before Ma Bell died and the telephone company's house calls ceased.

The men left, promising to return that afternoon to complete the job. The second time around I greeted them dressed in slick jeans tucked into high boots, a green turtleneck sweater, full makeup, and Jackie Kennedy's latest hairdo. Chatting comfortably while sharing coffee, I decided on a different spot in the kitchen for the ivory wall phone.

"But," one stammered as he pointed to my earlier site selection, "the lady who was here this morning wanted it over there."

"That was no lady, that was me."

His partner looked doubtful. "I thought she was your mother."

What can you say to that? I tipped them five bucks.

Nothing has changed in the ensuing thirty years. I still get better service when I'm well dressed, wearing makeup, and my hair is having a good day. I feel better, too.

Before painting a pretty picture on our faces, we need to prepare our less-than-elastic skin, our largest organ and, unlike our livers, very visible.

Nature covered us in skin, swathing us from head to toe like beautiful gift wrapping. We're cute little packages when we're delivered. Then just as with gift wrapping, our skin becomes flattened, spotted, faded, crumpled, and unraveled with use. That's putting it kindly. Some people save wrapping paper, folding it carefully, ironing out its wrinkles, recycling it. With such tender care their packaging can look as good as those covered in fresh paper. But no one ever said it would be easy.

I have reached an age where the only oily area left on my face is the bottom of my nose, a welcome oasis in a desert of dry skin. It's also the only spot where astringent is needed. Be discriminating with astringent. Don't use it on arid areas crying for cream. Anything placed, patted, or spread on dry skin should leave it feeling softer and smoother, or why bother? Moisturize your parched and thirsty body parts yearning to be refreshed. Apply your grease of choice twice a day to squeaky clean skin. Consider it as necessary as your daily change of underwear.

Skin Care Routine

IN THE MORNING

1. Wash your face. I like Dove unscented for sensitive skin, and I use a facecloth. There are other viable options: cleansing creams, lotions, expensive soaps, designed as part of an extensive skin care program. There is no one correct choice. Just make sure the skin is clean with no residue.

2. Apply astringent to oily areas. That step will close your pores and absorb any oil. I use witch hazel. It's natural, cheap, and lasts forever— I have only that one oily patch—and can be used for sundry bites and mysterious bumps. These bumps always burst through my skin when I'm going to a party. Oil-less ghosts of teenage pimples. They vanish as mysteriously as they appear, but never in time for the party.

3. Apply moisturizer liberally. Spread it upward and outward. Don't pull your skin down. Age and gravity don't need your help. Let your fingers fly over your face in upward movements. Be especially generous in the eye area and around the mouth. I use totally hypoallergenic moisturizer that is 100 percent fragrance free. I buy unscented deodorant, hair spray, toilet paper, tissues, detergent, and even fabric softener, so I certainly don't want my moisturizer to contain perfume. I've never understood the popularity of scented toilet paper or why anyone would want to blow her nose into a scented tissue. Scented cosmetics clash with each other and with any cologne you may be wearing. I guess I'm just an unscented woman.

BEFORE BEDTIME

1. Remove all makeup. I don't care how tired you are or how late it is, take it off—unless, of course, you're going to bed with a new man. That's the only acceptable excuse for sleeping in makeup. And be very careful. Just a little lip gloss and blush. Overnight mascara will stain your face, turning you into a haggard raccoon in the morning, not to mention what it will do to your or his pillowcase. I've used Pond's Cold Cream for over forty-five years. I've tried many more expensive cleansers and even herbal products, but they don't take it all off as effectively as good old reliable Pond's.

2. Once your face is washed or cleansed with your preferred product, use astringent where needed and apply night cream. Purchasing the latter can require a cosigned loan. Most night creams are more expensive than the monthly rent was for my first apartment. And since I slather the stuff all over my face and neck—all this cleaning and moisturizing should include the neck area—I'm always running out. But I found the right way to oil up for bed without going broke. Most cosmetic houses offer night creams, and some even deliver as promised—reducing the appearance of fine lines and wrinkles. Several years ago, *Dateline* debunked many cosmetic claims. Among them was one company's eighty-five-dollar-an-ounce caviar eggs "guaranteed" to make a fifty-year-old look thirty. Other companies' claims were equally exaggerated. I've always suspected that there isn't much difference between moisturizing lotions; *Dateline*'s investigation proved it. They found Vaseline Intensive Care Lotion at twenty-eight cents an ounce the best moisturizer and by the far the most economical. I switched to Vaseline Intensive Care that day.

The following Christmas when I visited my friend Doris, she commented on how good my skin looked. I picked up her giant-sized Vaseline Intensive Care, which she'd been using for decades on her body. "This is what I've been using on my face." Doris, a nurse by training and glamorous by birthright, who has always purchased the crème de la crème of cosmetics and moisturizers, started applying the body lotion to her face that very day.

Whatever product you choose, remember they're called night creams because you wear them while you're sleeping. Once you become used to the routine, you'll do all this, floss and Interplak your teeth, and be in the sack in fifteen minutes. Okay, twenty.

IN THE SHOWER OR TUB

I know some consider soap a dirty word, but I also use Dove to clean the old bod. Once a week, though twice would be better, I use a body sloughing cream in the shower to get rid of dead surface cells. Or try loofah gloves. They slough off dry skin and stimulate circulation. These loofahs are easy to use, come in bright colors, and are gentle to the skin. They're sold in department stores for under ten dollars.

Showers are quick, efficient, and the best place to wash your hair. You're in and out in ten minutes, you don't dry out your skin, and you get a mini massage from the water bouncing off your body. Sixty-four percent of Americans prefer a shower to a bath.

Yet I love a bubble bath where I can relax and read.

Betty Grable took a lot of on-screen bubble baths in those old movie musicals. In *Diamond Horseshoe* she even entertained a visitor. The bubbles covered the modesty requirement, while one of her famous legs was washed before our very eyes. She always wore her hair piled on top of her head . . . and full makeup. Sometimes I apply makeup, style my hair, hop in the tub, and wash from the neck down. The theory is I won't get my hair wet as I would in the shower and will emerge ready to dress. However, I suspect I'm still playing movie stars.

The psychological pleasures of the bath renew my spirit. There are several magic potions you can add to the water to enhance your soak. And it's a great way to feel sensual and beautiful, especially if you light candles tubside. Then you may wish to share the experience with a husband or very close friend.

After the shower or bath, apply body lotion generously; let it dry before dressing. If I'm going out, I apply makeup and blow-dry my hair while my thirsty body absorbs its daily dose of grease. I use the same Vaseline Intensive Care that I use on my face—the one marked for dry, sensitive skin. If I'm staying home, I saturate my feet, pull on old white socks, and let it all soak in overnight. The morning-after ritual includes changing the sheets.

TWICE A WEEK

Use a facial mask—Almay's Hydrating Mask for Dry Skin or Orlane Exfoliating Cream. I like Clinique's 7-Day Scrub. It's more gentle. Follow the directions on tube or jar, and avoid using around the eyes. The results are softer, smoother skin. I should probably apply a mask more often. Actually, there are many days that I look better wearing one!

DO FACE EXERCISES

1. To avoid a double chin: stand straight, pull your head up out of your neck, and then bend your chin to your chest. Next, stand tall, with head straight. Lunge your face forward. Stick out your tongue and try to touch your chin. Repeat eight times. Never perform this exercise in front of an audience.

2. To soften lines around mouth while lifting your cheeks: Open your mouth as wide as possible and grin as broadly as you can. Then go for a bigger grin. Hold for a count of ten. Repeat eight times.

3. To tone the eye area: Open your eyes as wide as possible. Lift your brows. Stare at an object across the room. Focus and hold the gaze for a count of ten. Lower your brows and close your eyes for a count of ten. Repeat eight times.

4. To help firm up sags and lines in your neck or to postpone their arrival, do this neck stretch: Stand tall with feet flat on the floor, tummy in, and head high. Turn your neck as far to the right as you can. Drop your head to your shoulder. Hold for a count of eight. Repeat the movement to the left. *Do not* strain. Then drop your head to your chest. Hold for a count of eight. Do these exercises slowly to achieve maximum benefit.

5. To lift those facial muscles a big smile is the best exercise. Your face flows in an upward motion. Repeat two hundred times a day.

FROM INSIDE OUT

Are eight cups of tea acceptable substitutes for the recommended eight glasses of water? A great gulper of liquids, water is not among my top ten drinks of choice.

Frazier's Jane Reeves in *Woman's World* credited liquids for her great skin. "Soups, teas, Popsicles, and skim milk" are imbibed daily. That's comforting. All of the above are on my top ten list. But I'm still working on my lack of water problem. I know that eight glasses a day flushes out our systems, and I don't want mine to back up.

Also working from inside out are vitamins. A, E, and C act as anti-oxidants. Vitamin A can be found in milk, yellow fruits, green and yellow veggies, and egg yolks. Oranges—80 percent water—are a wonderful source of vitamin C. And the B vitamins improve our nails, hair, vision, and even our brains—along with our skin. If we imbibe these vitamins, together with at least 1,200 milligrams of calcium fortified with vitamin D, every day, our skin and bones should hold together. Antioxidants quell free radicals, which age the skin by breaking down collagen and tissue. Those naughty free radicals are the result of sun, pollution, and smoking.

So swallow those vitamins and drink up—"Here's looking at you"—to stay foxy forever.

Home and Other Remedies

While raiding the refrigerator for skin-enhancing potables, forage for inexpensive beauty aids. What we're not eating could turn into cost-effective skin care, resulting in new looks for our fading faces.

• Whip up a mask of egg whites; it has the same results as cosmetic companies' masks but is much cheaper. You can use the yoke to condition your hair.

• Mash a papaya or mango (full of vitamin A) with a tablespoon of oatmeal and a tablespoon of chopped orange peel. Use to slough off dead cells and peeling or flaky dry skin. Just rub on moist skin, leave on for ten minutes, and then remove with warm water.

• Try cucumber slices to reduce bags or puffiness under the eyes. Lie down with feet elevated and place slices on eyes for ten minutes. Or try whole milk, not skim, to soothe red, scaly eyelids. Place milk-saturated pads on closed eyes for five to ten minutes, then rinse with cool water.

Don't use milk for puffy eyes. Try tea bags, my longtime remedy. Again lie down. Place cooled but still damp tea bags on your own bags for at least ten minutes. You'll get up looking ten years younger. Well . . . five, anyway.

Chronic dark circles and puffy lower lids are helped by sleeping on your back, so fluid doesn't build up, and by using cold compresses when you wake up. Our refrigerators can keep our compresses and creams cold while keeping our seldom used cosmetics crisp.

One beau, rummaging through my refrigerator for a Bud, discovered three out-of-date shades of nail polish and my teeth bleaching kit! This package included a container for my plastic dental impressions, which were used to hold the bleaching gel over my teeth. I never heard from him again— either because I had no beer or because he believed I had no teeth.

Teeth, yellowed with time, can be bleached back to white. A painless procedure once available only to the rich and famous is now available from your local dentist. Or in an abridged version, a bleaching kit can be purchased at your local drugstore. The dentist's process costs a lot more but is also more effective and does include those dental impressions to hold the bleaching gel in place. Either way, it's a home remedy. Store the gel in the refrigerator, and you can rewhiten when needed. Notice those TV and magazine ads that feature models over fifty—and sometimes sixty or seventy, and isn't that great? They may have wrinkles and an occasional jowl, but their teeth are always *white*! Now ours can be, too.

So What About Wrinkles?

We can wage war, but can we win? Do we really want to? Jane Fonda, my former *Password* playing partner, was quoted in the October 16, 1995, issue of *People* as saying, "Make friends with the aging process—and your wrinkles." Yeah, yeah. But some days that's easier said than done, Jane.

Why do we wrinkle? It's a natural aging process. Our older bodies produce less of two protein strands in the dermis, our lower layer of skin.

How to Avoid New Wrinkles

Don't smoke.

Drink lots of liquids.

Use sunscreen even in the winter and don't suntan (boy, am I sorry I ever did!).

Do face exercises daily.

Moisturize twice a day and add alpha hydroxy to your beauty routine.

Lose weight slowly.

Clean your face thoroughly and apply night cream before going to sleep.

These strands are elastin, which helps skin bounce back, and collagen, which forms our skin's foundation.

The following can help:

Alpha hydroxy acid (AHA), available as an over-the-counter cream, seems to smooth fine lines. It's one of the cosmetic companies' dream ingredients, but it's rooted in nature, garnered from lemons, apples, and passion fruit. You can buy alpha hydroxy acid lotion at the drugstore and apply it straight from the bottle for about five or six dollars—far less than the department stores' high-priced beauty creams.

Retin A stimulates production of new collagen and elastin fibers. It helps erase wrinkles by peeling off dead cells and making way for new healthy ones. Don't even think about Retin A if you're still going out in the sun! My early boomer friend Ellen Johnson has been using it for a few years, and her fair skin looks sensational. And so did the glowing skin of several sixty-plus interviewees. It's a good idea to check with your dermatologist before using any new product.

Deep acid peels contain high concentrations of trichloroacetic acid. It is applied to the skin, blisters form, and healing takes a couple of weeks. Many women are opting for a face peel. Not me. No way! I once watched a coworker go through this procedure; it was a horror show. Instead of weeks, it took months before her red, raw face healed. And for the first three or four days she could barely walk. I will say, when she did heal, her skin was as clear as a child's. Of course this gal was only thirty-five. Results and discomfort can vary dramatically.

Collagen injections are costly but effective. Expect to pay from $300 to $800 for a ten- to fifteen-minute procedure. The good news: The patient's own collagen will kick in and fill in the wrinkles, allowing a longer time span between shots—if you don't go bankrupt first.

Remember: A man's morning mirror image is as good as he will get to look all day long. What a ghastly thought! But Wonderful Older Women have an arsenal of weapons to aid us in life's daily scrimmages: the ammunition in our cosmetics bags. There's not a face that won't become more alive with a touch of color—even in the world's worse-lighted mirror. Subtle camouflage, not war paint.

Makeup: Don't leave home without it. Please turn the page and Paint Your Wagon!

Paint Your Wagon

"High maintenance," my niece groans, checking the clock. She's grumbling about the amount of time I spend getting ready. "What *are* you doing in there?" "In there" is the bathroom, and what I'm doing is putting on my makeup.

A slow starter, I've heard variations of that question since I was a teenager and my father wanted me out of the bathroom. He'd say to my mother, "What in God's name could your daughter be doing in there for nearly an hour?" Actually, for me an hour could be considered a short overhaul.

Decades later my French friend, Janine, would say to another of her houseguests, "Noreen has the world's longest toilette. She won't be out of there for ages. Why don't you use the other bathroom?"

Unfortunately, I haven't significantly improved on my toilette time with age, but I have shaved off thirty minutes.

For years, if I showered, washed and dried my hair, used hot rollers, slathered cream on face and body, sipped two or three cups of tea, applied full makeup, and slipped into my clothes, my total toilette could take up to ninety minutes. That daily routine often meant getting up at dawn to put my best face forward for my audience and get on the road. Today the total picture runs about an hour. And when I eliminate the makeup and hairstyling, I can be ready in fifteen minutes. Since I work at home alone, I'm all revved up in relatively short order, with a naked face, dressed in rag bags, and praying no one drops by.

I realize that even though my current bathroom lighting is flattering, I don't want to spend too much time in there, giving myself grief while checking out any new wrinkle or looking for falling hair. The good news is that my vision has faded some along with my face. Also, I'm well aware that an obsession with wanting to look as young as possible for as long as possible can steal several hours from a productive day. And I know that being foxy forever is an attitude, not a paint job. However, I also know that total resignation—ignoring a regular beauty routine and not putting on any makeup—can turn a WOW into a prune face.

Makeup in moderation is very much in vogue. There's never been a better beauty climate for growing into a WOW; looking natural is the way to go. Thank God! We've all shuddered at the sight of an old gal with bright red circles savagely rubbed into her sagging cheeks. A really bad paint job. Color can be our best friend if we use it judiciously.

Check out the makeup and hairstyles on women in the public eye, Wonderful Older Women whom you admire, women over fifty like Susan Sarandon, Diane Keaton, Hillary Clinton, and Diane Sawyer. Sawyer gets an A+ across the board: understated makeup, simple hairstyle, and classic clothes. And the women over sixty like Mary Tyler Moore, Elizabeth Dole, Diahann Carroll (on stage playing the psychiatrist in *Agnes of God*, she was the most beautiful woman I'd ever seen), Carol Burnett, and Maya Angelou. And those who are foxy forever like Barbara Walters, Lauren Bacall, Angela Lansbury, and Dr. Ruth Westheimer.

Not too long ago women over fifty walked a thin line between looking overpainted and garish or looking like an unpainted, rather stern Mother Superior. Many liquid and cream bases were too heavy to apply with a light touch, and with the foundation caking and cracked, the rest of the makeup appeared artificial. For some of us a bare face can still be beautiful. However, as a woman whose natural skin tone is greige, a little color goes a long way. For most of us, a light foundation is the cornerstone of building a better face than the one we woke up with. Whether a face is too sallow, too ruddy, too pale, or too blotchy, the right base can color-correct and give it a healthy glow.

A New Century Calls for a New Look

Start by cleaning out your cosmetic bag. We throw away old paint, discard expired medicines, and replace used sponges that harbor bacteria, but some of us have eye shadow older than our firstborn. Toss out all blue shadow, black mascara, or harsh black eyebrow pencils, as well as any too matte, and too dry or too old lipsticks.

Then consider buying a bunch of really good makeup brushes in all different sizes and shapes, structured for the various areas where you'll be applying makeup—eyelids, brows, lips, cheeks. For all over your face, use a big fat powder brush. You deserve to have a clean sweep across your new millennium face. And an old makeup brush, like an old paintbrush, clumps up; its bristles stick together, fail to absorb the fresh paint, and prevent a smooth application of color.

Taking a foxy forever approach to find a way to put our best faces forward, I interviewed cosmetic consultant and beauty expert Bridgit Fitzgerald, who has twenty years of experience at upscale department stores developing special makeup techniques for women over fifty. In a private consultation Bridgit shared her secrets and provided solutions for dry skin, lines, wrinkles, and uneven skin tone, as well as step-by-step instructions for painting a WOW face.

Millennium Makeover

Step One: Concealer. Apply a yellow-tone concealer sparingly around the full eye area and directly under the bottom lip. Blend thoroughly but gently. Believe it or not, a yellow tone gives a calm, rested look to the skin and works well for a wide range of skin tones. Bridgit and her staff use Lancôme's Maquicomplet Correcteur, a complete coverage concealer, in their makeup demonstrations.

Step Two: Base. Apply a light-diffusing liquid or cream foundation to match your skin tone. Bridgit prefers liquid because it looks more natural if applied and blended correctly. Start out with an amount no larger than a dime. Use a sponge or your fingertips. Apply to your

T-zone—across your forehead and down the center of your nose—and blend outward. While moisturizer should be applied in an upward motion, lifting any sags as you go along, in the application of base, use an outward and downward stroke so you don't raise any fine hairs. Bridgit advises using a base that contains sunscreen as well as a light diffuser. She recommends Teint Lift Eclat—Essential Firming Makeup by Chanel or Lucidity by Estée Lauder.

Step Three: Powder. Apply loose powder. "Should you do that even if your skin is really dry and you have lines?" I asked.

"Absolutely!" Bridgit said. "Bobbi Brown's powder makes people look ten years younger! And powder should be applied with a large powder brush. I like Trish McEvoy's brushes. Give the face a light dusting and avoid the eye area. Loose powder allows the rest of your makeup to blend smoothly; otherwise, your blush goes on like spackle!"

Step Four: Blush. Take your blush powder brush and dip it into your blush. (See what I mean about investing in a full set of makeup brushes? We have to have the right tools!) Sweep the brush over the blush and smooth it over your cheeks, nose, and forehead—everywhere the sun would kiss your face. A smidgen on your eyelids wakes you up and makes your eyes sparkle. Bridgit said Bobbi Brown's Sand Pink is the perfect blush for cheeks that have lost their bloom.

When you've completed this step, your face is primed. You're ready to move on to the eyes, the mirrors to our souls.

Step Five: Mascara. Apply several coats of mascara. Many makeup artists and most of us civilians apply mascara after we've applied eye shadow and liner. However, Bridgit explained that putting on mascara at this juncture allows us to remove those little dots of mascara that somehow always wind up on our lids without smudging our eye shadow or liner. And if needed, one last coat of mascara can be added—carefully—when makeup application is finished.

Step Six: Eye shadow. Using a light shade, cover the entire upper lid area from lash to brow, Bridgit advises. "This gives you a good canvas to work on." Then with your shader brush, apply the pale shadow to any dark areas in the inside corners next to your eyes. I was amazed at how that trick "opened up" my eyes and how wide awake I looked.

Matte neutral shades like taupe, pale gray, and heather are best for contouring. Some pink shadows can make an eye look sore or swollen. Avoid frost and shimmer, which only highlight creases, puffiness, or dryness.

Using a shadow brush, apply the neutral shade along the center crease, from the middle of the eye out. Exactly how you apply the shadow depends on the shape of your eye. Visit a cosmetic consultant at a better department store. He or she will do a makeover free of charge. Ask lots of questions. What about all these color choices? What shades go together? Which are best for your eyes? Should shadows ever match your clothes? How can you turn your daytime look into evening drama?

Step Seven: Eyeliner. Use a fine liner such as Chanel's shadow liner brush, and smudge as you apply so you don't have a harsh line. Lancôme's Artline is like a felt-tip pen and comes in a great color for older faces: *grappe*. This shade makes the eyes sparkle, and with its plum undertones, it's not as harsh as black and won't make the eyes look red as many of the browns do.

Step Eight: Eyebrows. Bridgit stressed the importance of natural-looking brows. "They frame the face!" Dip an eyebrow brush lightly in a soft powder and apply, following your natural brow line. If your brows are plucked away, go easy on the pencil; it can be harsh and aging as well as dated. If you do use a pencil—Brigit recommends Chanel Precision Brow Definer—feather the line with a brush and a bit of shadow. Blend and then brush and feather. The result should look like hair, not a penciled-in hard line.

Step Nine: Minimizing wrinkles with a magic golden wand! Use Yves St. Laurent's Touche Eclat/Radiant Touch. This mini miracle is applied after all your other makeup except lipstick. Put it on anywhere you see a line. It deflects light and seems to lift away your lines, resulting in a radiant appearance. Spread from the bottom of your nose into the lines around your nostrils, then fill in those deep puppet lines that run from your mouth to your chin, and all around your mouth before you apply lipstick. Blend with your fingertips.

Bridgit said, "My mother's always asking me to bring her that golden wand that takes all the wrinkles away." Her mom is seventy and looks great.

Step Ten: Lipstick. Apply a lip cream and let it dry for a half hour before applying lipstick. If your lips are anywhere near as dry as mine were, you'll take Bridgit's advice: Do it first, and by the time you get the rest of your face on, your lips will be ready. (My own tip: I use an inexpensive Revlon lip base that does double duty as an eyeshadow base.)

Use a lip liner. Fill in both the top and bottom lip with the liner. I learned something new there! Use a creamy coral-color lipstick. Bridgit told me, "Brown, neutral, and blue-red lipstick shades are aging on older faces. The vast majority of mature women look best in coral. Its warmth adds a glow. Chanel's Rich Coral and Jubilee and Yves St. Laurent's #52 are good choices for mature faces." I told her that I prefer WOW to mature.

If you want to shape your jawline, contour your cheeks, or cover brown age spots, a cosmetic consultant can be a WOW's best friend. It's our chance to reaffirm our assets, cover up our flaws, and emerge as the best we can be. You'll learn a lot, and when the makeup artist has finished, you'll walk away looking great. And you don't have to buy a thing, though you probably will! I know I did. And even allowing for inflation, Leonardo da Vinci's paintbrushes couldn't have cost anywhere near as much as the three I bought!

Though I had received an "A" for the makeup I walked in wearing, after my makeover I said, "Wow!" And why not? This new look totaled over $500! The cosmetics cost $314.92 and, though we hadn't even touched the tips of all the brushes recommended for "correct" application of the myriad of makeup, the brushes we did use ran well over $200.

"God, Bridgit," I said. "If a woman were to buy all the cosmetics you used on me today, she'd spend a small fortune—and that's not even counting the cost of the creams and other skin care products you've recommended." I thought about how effective my inexpensive drugstore products' skin care routine had always been. "What about buying some comparable cosmetics at a drugstore?"

People are paying for packaging, I kept thinking. And makeup has the highest markup percentage of any retail product.

"I might not be able to find a replacement for everything—there's probably no magic wand or I'd have known about it—but their stuff wouldn't be a quarter of the price of these designer brands."

Bridgit Fitzgerald smiled. "A cashmere sweater made in China will not compare to one from Scotland."

"Well, if a woman wants to look great but doesn't want to float a face-improvement loan to cover the cost, which of these cosmetics would be most important?"

She didn't hesitate. "Don't skimp on concealer, base, powder, or brushes. And no woman over fifty should face the world without the magic wand wrinkle deflector.

I thanked her for a fun and informative afternoon and headed to CVS, my local drugstore chain, for a cosmetic cost analysis. While I then used—and still do—Clinique's soft finish base, I knew that many of the drugstore's cosmetics worked really well for me. And at the very least I could save myself and others a bundle on lipstick, lip liner, eye shadow, and eyeliner. And I knew I could buy all the brushes I needed for under thirty dollars. Good ones, too.

All the drugstore products worked beautifully, and it was a huge savings. However, you might want to treat yourself as well as your wrinkles and lines. Go ahead, splurge on Yves St. Laurent's Radiant Touch. It is a magic wand, and I need one!

Getting Ready for Prime Time

Whether we opt for a $99 discount drugstore face or a $500 department store face, the real secret for a natural look is not only choosing the right foundation but applying it correctly. Matte, sheer, light-diffusing, oil-free, cream, stick, or liquid? Which is right for you? How can you be sure that your cover-up will look natural? What's the best way to blend? Should a sponge be used? A cosmetic consultant can select a foundation with the texture and consistency that's best for your complexion and do your makeup that day, but when you're on your own, here are some helpful hints for buying and applying the perfect base.

BASE BASICS

Neither you nor anyone else should be aware that you're wearing it. Don't use too much moisturizer before applying base. If you do, the base will feel heavy and look too shiny. A greasy or heavy result defeats a foundation's purpose: to enhance your skin tone. If your skin is oily—I should be so fortunate—use moisturizer only on your dry skin areas. If your skin is dry, let moisturizer sit for a few minutes and then blot before applying base.

Which foundation is the perfect finish for you? A light-diffusing formula that reflects light away from lines and creases can be found in bases ranging from sheer to medium coverage and can be either oil-free or moisturizing. Most Wonderful Older Women should select the ones that indicate moisture rather than oil-free on their labels. These foundations often have "illuminating" on their labels, too. Almay Time Off Age Soothing Makeup is an inexpensive but fine finish. So is Revlon Age Defying Makeup. I'm a big fan of light-diffusing bases as long as they contain moisturizers.

If you're interested in a moisturizing base, and most of us with dry skin are, you can find it in sheer to full coverage. These bases offer both moisture and a dewy finish all day long. Clinique Balanced Makeup Base—I like this one a lot—and Prescriptives Makeup+ are two moisturizing foundations.

A stick foundation, such as Max Factor's Pan Stick Ultra Creamy Makeup, offers full coverage but may be too heavy for any WOW; it proved too thick and masklike for my dry skin. Some women have used it for years and like its "velvet" finish. This stick can be applied judiciously on scars and other spots. Bobbi Brown's Stick was more expensive but worth it. The finish is fantastic. And Oprah carries it in her purse. But my skin is *so* dry, I use it only for spot coverage.

Cream bases loaded with moisturizers provide full coverage and are designed for older, dry, lined, or wrinkled faces. Mine certainly qualifies! However, I found cream coverage far too heavy no matter how small an amount I spread over my skin. Ultima II Ultimate Coverage and indeed it is—is a popular cream foundation.

Choosing the correct color.   Match your skin tone. Too dark a tone can look muddy and streaked. Too light can make you look ill. Lana Rizzo, another makeup artist, told me, "If you have a yellow undertone, as I do, go with it. Choose a base, blush, and eye shadow to flatter your natural skin color."

In any upscale department store the cosmetic consultants represent many ethnic backgrounds and will work with you to choose the correct shade. Remember that the lighting at any cosmetic counter's mirror is very flattering. And often, so is the consultant.

When you're heading to a drugstore's cosmetics aisle, stash a mirror in your tote bag, and before you buy, carry the bottle of base that you fancy over to the window and hold it next to your neck near your jawline. Daylight may be harsh, but it's accurate and usually far better than most drugstores' fluorescent overhead lighting.

If you're debating between a lighter and a darker shade, opt for the lighter one. Or buy both and create your own color!

When applying, remember: Less is more.   You can use a slightly damp sponge. Many experts say it provides the smoothest application. I prefer my fingers, spreading a dime-size amount of foundation gently over my face. But stop at your jawline. If you've brought home the right color, your base should match your neck. You never want to apply base to your neck.

A light touch and lots of blending will result in a sheer, natural appearance. Attempting to cover up blemishes or age spots will only look heavy-handed. That's why we have concealer, to be strategically applied after moisturizer but before the base. And if you have freckles, they should be showing through the base; otherwise, the coverage is too heavy.

A very light dusting of powder will set the base, but let the foundation dry before brushing on the powder. Rely on pressed powder, which looks cakey and heavy, only as a touch-up—for example, if your nose gets shiny during the day—and apply as seldom as possible. Blotting with a tissue or one of those little cosmetic companies' blotting papers is a much better idea.

Mastering these base basics will have you primed to face the day.

BLUSHING BEAUTY

A good blush should leave you looking as if you're blushing just a bit. Clinique Blushwear's Blush is a great shade for women of color. The cream rouge consistency reminds me of what my mother used fifty years ago, and the formula still works. Smooth and easy to work with, it is available in shades to enhance every skin tone.

THE EYES HAVE IT

Drugstore eye makeup is, in my opinion, better than the department store's costly counterparts. You can't beat Maybelline. *Glamour* endorsed its new Wonder Curl mascara; however, I prefer Great Lash, tried and true for decades. L'Oréal's Voluminous has a smooth application that thickens without clumps. Almay's One Step isn't, but it does make your lashes look fantastic.

THE SHADOWS I KNOW

Any Maybelline matte neutral color finish (you should avoid the dark plums and bright blues) is not only a great buy but a great product. And Cover Girl's Pro Shadow is a steal. Maybelline's Line Works will line your eyes in style for a great price. So there's no need to pay big bucks for great eyes.

SLICK LIPS

Following Bridgit's advice, coral is the color for most Wonderful Older Women. I mix and match to create my own shade. I use and recommend Revlon's Moondrop Chinaglaze Red, topped with Maybelline's Moisture Whip Strawberry Cream, and glossed over with Cover Girl's Lip Slicks.

If you're ready to go for broke, I really liked the Chanel lipstick color Rich Coral. Its warm tones will light up your face, but its matte finish was too dry for me.

Most inexpensive lipsticks contain the same ingredients as the expensive ones; you're paying for the fancy packaging. Selecting the right shade and texture—look for smooth moisture—is more important than a designer label. Drugstore lipstick works as well as those that cost five times as much.

Here are some more tips for smooth lips that won't bleed into those tiny lines around the mouth: Buff your lips with a damp toothbrush to remove dry skin. Then shape, outline, and fill in your lips with a liner, and apply a coating of creamy lipstick. If your lipstick still bleeds—as mine would if I didn't use the following tourniquet—apply a moisturizing base. Vaseline is fine. Let it dry, and then outline your lips, filling in only the insides and using a dewy, non-matte, easy-to-spread lipstick such as Maybelline's Moisture Whip, and top with gloss.

Selecting lipstick shades that whiten your teeth.   If your teeth are tinged with yellow, avoid blue-based reds, fuchsia (a hard color to wear anyway), plums, and pink tones. These cool colors clash with yellow and make the teeth look worse than ever. Try warm tones to take the yellow away. Once again, coral is the color of choice to make teeth look whiter.

Or Just Go Ahead and Bleach Those Former Pearly Whites

Several years ago I woke up one morning—or so it seemed—to discover my colors had changed. I was no longer a spring, summer, or even fall. Dead of winter would be a more apt seasonal description. My complexion had acquired a gray, pasty tone, my roots had turned from silver to stark white, framing my face in an unbecoming fashion, and my teeth appeared dingy, a yellow-beige that if found on a patient's skin would have been diagnosed as jaundice. Knowing I could color-correct my hair (please see next chapter) and change my foundation to a warmer tone, I thought first things first, and made an emergency appointment at the dentist.

The bleaching process involved two visits, having impressions made of my upper and lower teeth, and a fifteen-minute lesson from the dentist, including watching a video, on the techniques of successful whitening. On the second visit I received plastic covers, custom-designed for my teeth; I filled these with the bleaching gel and then slipped them in place over my teeth to be left on overnight. After wearing these plastic caps to bed for three weeks, my teeth were much whiter. At a cost of $300. I still keep the gel and the caps in the refrigerator, and once in a blue moon—or yellow funk—I reapply. (This was the unappealing package that sent the refrigerator-rummaging date running home.)

Today there are more options. You can pay the dentist, or you can purchase a complete kit at the drugstore and bleach your teeth at home—maybe on the same night you color your hair.

Facing the Future

Whatever you decide is your right look is the look that's right for you. From au natural to a well-covered finish, the face you present to the world should make a statement about the WOW who is behind the facade.

Chapter 6

Silver Threads
Among the Gold

From hair to eternity. My months of research into how best to treat our crowning glory has reinforced my belief that a woman's mane can be both a bane and a blessing. Long, lustrous hair represents femininity to most men. An image of copious locks spread across a pillow sells everything from romance novels to shampoo. Bouncing hair grazing a young woman's shoulders as she dashes across a grassy meadow toward a handsome man's waiting arms has become a television commercial cliché. The message: Hair is an aphrodisiac. The more of it you have, the more womanly you are. Long, lush tresses evoke sexual desire in men. While you and I may know this is nonsense, many men—and too many women—have bought into this Rapunzel spin.

Older men's attitudes have been colored by many decades of accepting this long-hair-equals-sex-appeal myth. Vanna White won her job on *Wheel of Fortune* because she reminded the show's creator, Merv Griffin, of his film idol, Rita Hayworth. Vanna—at Griffin's strong suggestion—copied Hayworth's long, sexy, forties hairstyle for years. When White finally decided to cut it short, Griffin was rumored to be disappointed.

"We were cute when we were supposed to be," explained Diane Dowling Dufour, a former successful photographic model and Aquacade professional swimmer, now my dear friend, a wise WOW, and a beauty consultant to her peers. "It's okay to want to be chic, attractive, even beautiful, but forget cute. Just because a pageboy was your signature style through your teens, twenties, and thirties, don't assume it still suits you in your fifties. And as for a ponytail, no matter how bad a hair day you're having, just forget about it!"

Chances are, if you're over fifty and your hair is long enough to pull back into a ponytail, it's too long.

Yes, but I look good in long hair. There are exceptions. Lauren Bacall—over seventy and a definite WOW—has worn the same simple, skimming-the-shoulders style since the fifties when she snipped her trademark forties long hair. Simple is the secret of her hairstyle's enduring success. My personal heroine, the late Jacqueline Kennedy Onassis, wore her hair long enough to pull back—though never in a ponytail—and I believe Jackie could be considered the most influential fashion icon of the twentieth century. There are many elegant Wonderful Older Women who choose to wear their long locks in French twists, chignons, or in crowns atop their heads—and look regal.

Too often, however, straggly hair falling below the shoulders can turn an otherwise attractive fifty-plus woman into a haggard-looking witch or a cartoon character. Some of you may recall Gravel Gertie, the wife of B. O. Plenty, in Dick Tracy comic strip. And some of you, like me, may have noticed the cascading curls of a woman walking in front of you, only to have her turn around and you're staring in amazement at the face of an old lady.

Yet too short a style can sometimes be worse than too long. We don't want to look too stark or too mannish. And it's sad but true that most women over fifty are too old to wear a boyish bob. A WOW might want to strike a happy medium, finding a flattering hairstyle that's long enough to soften and short enough to be chic. The biggest challenge a WOW has when choosing the right hairstyle is how to look classic but current.

Choose a Classic and Current Haircut
That Flatters Your Face

The very rich are different from you and me. They have better hairstylists. I went to Great Lengths, an upscale Washington, D.C., salon, to chat with one of those stylists.

Chris Berg has been a hairstylist since 1971, though looking at her slim figure and chic short blond hair, that hardly seems possible. In 1990, Chris opened her own salon in the downtown section of D.C. and today has eighteen employees and a large clientele, including some famous Washington faces.

"When cutting and styling an older woman's hair, do you agree with the conventional wisdom that shorter is younger?" I asked Chris.

Her answer surprised me. "That's often good advice, but depending on the size and shape of the woman's face and the texture of her hair, I find almost as often that hair framing an older client's face will soften her lines and flatter her features. I take into consideration the whole person, including the head size and body size. Too short a hairstyle can make a very tall woman look like a pinhead."

"So, Chris, what percentage of your clients over fifty opt for medium to long hair?"

"Seventy percent of them wear their hair no longer than two inches below the ear."

"Why?" If many older women would look better with more hair, I wanted to know why a staggering 70 percent chose a short cut.

"Because it's easy to style," Chris said. "These are busy women, with neither the time nor the inclination to fuss with their hair on a daily basis."

Chris sported and recommends a short style but cut with long layers on top to give it shape and some swing. "It's feminine as well as flattering to most faces."

"What about an equally flattering longer style?"

"Consider a mid-length style, maybe to the chin, and layered and tucked behind the ears. It looks great on most women."

I nodded, knowing that the style Chris was describing is extremely popular. Indeed, it's the current coiffure of choice for many female TV news anchors.

Chris continued, "Tucking the hair behind the ears results in fewer vertical lines, deemphasizing those drag-down vertical lines we all develop as we age. Depending on the front of the cut—bangs or lifted up off the forehead—this style can be worn with almost any shape face."

"But can a WOW wear her hair long and look chic?" I asked. "Or isn't that a realistic goal? Are our longhaired days behind us?"

"Long straight hair—Cher hair, another seventies style that's in vogue again—really emphasizes those vile vertical lines, pulling older faces down toward the floor."

"How about an upsweep?"

"Loose and smooth looks much younger." Chris shrugged. "Up generally looks mature."

"Even the French twist?" I was thinking a twist may not be current, but it is a classic and certainly smooth.

"That's a style a few women still do favor," Chris said without much enthusiasm. She did concede, however, that the twist remains a classic.

How to Have Your Hair Cut to Make It Appear Fuller

At birth, 100 percent of a baby's scalp is covered with hair follicles. By the time that baby reaches fifty, some of those hair follicles have closed down and the hair produced is thinner. On average, by the age of fifty, 50 percent of our hair is gone. This is okay, according to Dr. John Wolf, a dermatologist at Baylor College of Medicine. If we're careful, the remaining 50 percent should be more than enough.

But while some Wonderful Older Women will retain thick locks through their next incarnation, others suffer here and now from much more hair loss than the 50 percent average—even some highly visible TV personalities.

Chris and I discussed a very famous WOW television star, one of the many who wears that ubiquitous mid-length hairdo with bangs and tucked behind the ears. I said, "You can see the bald spots through the teasing when she bends forward and the overhead lights shine down on her crown."

"She'd be better off with shorter hair," Chris said. "For thinning hair, a close cut above the ears will lift up the rest of your hair. The shorter the hair is around the edges, the more the top layers are pushed up to make them appear fuller and thicker."

If you want to infuse short- to medium-length limp, thin hair with more body, a chin-length, lightly layered bob can do the trick and create an illusion of fullness. Or root lifting could be the route to take. On a wet head, rub in a tiny amount of a volume-increasing gel such as Volumax, which also adds shine, and comb it through the hair, starting at the roots. Be sure to cover all strands. Allow the hair to partly dry, then use your fingers, not a brush, as you blow-dry, lifting individual sections of hair up and away from the scalp. Smooth the outside hair strands with a natural-bristle brush. Spritz lightly. Too much spray will drag your hair right back down again.

Layering is one way to add volume, but many women have trouble styling a layered look at home. Chris's suggestion: "Just use a blow-dryer beginning with the roots. A very little bit of round brushing, maybe ten minutes, will complete the look, and the ends will fall into place." The right style can camouflage thin spots. Fluff bangs; use a curling iron or a large electric roller to achieve the appearance of volume, and then spread them out to cover too-high foreheads or bare temple areas. If it's the crown that's sparse, gently tease and then spray judiciously. You don't want the hairs to clump. And don't sit directly under television wattage lightbulbs.

Finally, an upsweep can be the perfect solution for thin hair. Even with male-pattern baldness, there's plenty of hair left on the sides and back of the head. If your hair is long, you can gather it all up, roll it into a twist, and then tease the top a tad. Everyone will think you have tons of thick hair.

Two of my foxy forever friends have complained of thinning hair for the last decade, but both have the problem areas well covered, styling their tresses so effectively that no one would ever suspect. Their hair always looks wonderful, and both of them attribute their successful cover-ups to great haircuts.

The right hair stylist who cuts creatively and works with her client's needs can be a WOW's best long-term investment.

Big Hair Is Out and Flat Hair Is In

The good news is that a WOW with fine, straight hair has never been more in style. And a WOW with strands to spare should never wear any style remotely resembling passé mall hair.

Celebrities with classic cuts include Diane Sawyer and Cokie Roberts. These two classy-from-top-to-bottom women will also be featured later, in the chapter on fashion. Hillary Clinton, after years of experimentation, has found a signature hairstyle that would look great on many other Wonderful Older Women. And while it may be a tad too teased, Elizabeth Dole's hair always looks politically correct.

How to Condition Your Crowning Glory

"Hair gets old like the rest of the body," Chris Berg said.

With my naturally porous, frequently colored hair, currently suffering from terminal dryness, I asked Chris what she could suggest as a quick fix. Again her answer surprised me.

"Look for a stylist who wants to be involved in the long-term health maintenance of your hair, a stylist who can offer ongoing prescriptive recommendations and design a treatment plan based on the best reconstructors required for the individual client's needs."

"So there's no panacea?"

"Patience." Chris smiled. "Often, instant repair products only mask the real problem."

I ran my fingers through my dry, frizzy hair. "What would this treatment consist of?" Instant shine products had made my hair look and feel better, but only temporarily. They never did get to the root of the problem.

"I use Redken products and Tiger Reconstructor by Wayne Grund—reconstructors that add protein, making chemical processes as well as conditioning processes work better."

"You mean if my dry hair had long-term reconstruction treatments, my future coloring process and conditioners would be more effective? Is this a prescription plan for better hair?"

"Exactly. A stylist's philosophy of hair care has never been so important." Chris explained: "Using today's advanced technology and a close monitoring of the state of the client's hair health, a stylist actually can both perm and color with very little damage if that is what the client wants or needs. Results look and feel great. But any chemical process can compromise the hair, the goal is to compromise it as little as possible."

For permanent improvements work with your hairstylist. A WOW who is on a budget, like me, can buy the prescribed Redken products at a beauty supply shop and do her own hair reconstruction work at home.

If your hair still needs an instant repair on occasion, the following quick fixes perform magic:

- Pro-Vitamin E Instant Repair: Two dollops of this gel cover the entire head. Use before styling. Smooths and shines instantly.
- Keihl's Silk Groom: Use your fingers to spread this moisturizing styling lotion through your hair to get rid of frizz and add shine.
- Aveda Pure-Fume Brilliant Hair Spray: The name says it all and, fortunately, it's far quicker to apply than to pronounce.
- Paul Mitchell's The Shine: Pricey but effective. Spray on dry hair before or after styling, and see it shine.

How to Tame That Wild Mane or Enjoy Being a Wild Woman

Flat hair is in fashion for now, but would you really want to control that curly top?

Consider the following Katharine Hepburn remarks about her style and her wild mane, as quoted in the July 1995 issue of *In Style* magazine: "I like to look as if I didn't give a damn. I think you should pretend you don't care . . . but it's the most outrageous pretense. I said to Garbo once, 'I bet it takes us longer to look as if we hadn't made any effort than it does for someone else to come in beautifully dressed.' I don't care a rap how I look, though I do wash my hair every night. It's harder to have a good-looking messy hairdo than a neat one. It's got to be messy just right."

With wonderful, thick, stubborn hair, the best control is a great cut. At home, wash, let dry naturally, and accept the frizzes. Or blow-dry, apply any of the instant shiners, and use large Velcro rollers at the crown and the sides for a somewhat smoother look. Don't try to make your hair appear totally flat. Why would you? Other Wonderful Older Women would trade their thin hair for your thick tresses in a New York millisecond.

Color to Dye For

It has been said that only in America do children believe that women become blonder as they grow older. If you opt to dye or bleach—and I've done both in various decades—watch out: Artificial must be natural or at least look natural.

No one is platinum at fifty. Unless you want to shout "bleached blonde," only tint two shades lighter than your original color. You can always add highlights. An ash or honey tone is more believable than a pale champagne or strawberry blond.

Whether you go lighter or darker, what you don't want is uniform color. Not only will it look dull, it will look dyed. There are several shade gradations in any head of virgin hair.

If your chestnut hair has turned dark and dull, don't decide to be a blonde. Lighten and brighten, but retain—or aim to return to—those warm brown tones. Natural-looking shades of brown may be better than blond for a brunette's skin tones. Besides, brown is now the hottest trend in hair coloring. Don't dye your hair black. It not only looks unreal but hard. Going to extremes—too light or too dark—will accentuate imperfections and age any face.

Try hair color swatches held next to your skin before deciding

While a hair salon may be the best place to dye or bleach, coloring in the comfort of your own home can be safe, simple, effective, and inexpensive. Chris suggests, "It may be a good idea to start with salon coloring so you know what to look for."

L'Oréal and Clairol, the masters of the color-at-home game, have developed products on a par with any salon. Of course, a professional colorist has more experience. But L'Oréal's Excellence Creme's pastelike consistency emulates salon products, adheres better than its liquid competition, and can be applied straight from the tube. And the results live up to its name.

GOING FOR THE GRAY

During my long day at Greatlengths, the best-looking woman I saw—with by far the sharpest, shortest style—sported a headful of glorious gray hair. When I told this silver fox how wonderful I thought she looked, she said, "It's so simple!"

And of course it was! Going back to natural could be the answer for your hair's future. No dyes, no perms, nothing but a smart cut once a month. The color is a gift from Mother Nature. Check out the growth at your roots. Your natural gray might look GREAT.

Extensions and Wigs

Attaching an extension to lengthen your locks or just to add volume, trendy among Generation Xers, works just as well for a WOW, and it can be a snap. There's a tiny metal comb hidden inside each hairpiece. You place the comb in your own hair, as close to the scalp as possible, and then snap it in. These extensions come in various sizes, from a small strand, to cover a bare spot, to a long fall, which can be twisted into an upsweep.

For serious hair loss resulting from illness or alopecia, a wig may be the answer. Actress Shirley Jones demonstrates how wonderful a wig can be. Natural hair is more expensive, but some synthetics are blended to look and feel like the real thing. You'll never have another bad hair day!

I wish every WOW great hair every day!

Climb Every Mountain

Wonderful Older Women realize that remaining foxy forever requires putting a little movement in our lives. We may never again see buns of steel—in my case they were always more like gelatin anyway—but we can become fit and semi-firm and, as a bonus, enjoy an attitude adjustment.

Thirty to forty minutes of exercise four days a week can keep us healthy, energized, and standing tall and straight. Time well spent, I'd say. And while a journey of a thousand miles begins with the first step, we really don't even need to leave home. But if your video workout tape or that lonely ride on your exercise bike has left you bored and not burning off fat, it's probably because you're no longer motivated by what you'd thought would be your final toning and tightening solution.

Maybe like most of us, when left to your own devices, you'd rather do the laundry, read a book, eat a Healthy Choice ice cream sandwich, or call your mother-in-law or even that woman your son thinks he wants to marry.

Still, the chances are awfully good, as Johnny Mathis sang, that you started an exercise program. But several of you, including me, might also admit to many false starts.

The number of people over fifty-five with health club memberships more than doubled between 1987 and 1997, according to a survey by the International Health, Racquet and Sportsclub Association. And the women over sixty-five averaged more exercise time at the clubs than their male counterparts. Most of the women I interviewed who were between fifty and sixty said that they were currently engaged in some sort of regular exercise, but the numbers dropped for those between sixty and seventy. Those women should be exercising! According to the January 12, 1999, issue of the *New York Times*, the *Journal of the American Geriatric Society* found that one-third of people over sixty-five fall at least once a year, many of them incurring injuries such as broken hips that may never properly heal. Experts believe these falls can be caused by a reduced sense of balance. Balancing exercises should be included in every aging woman's fitness plan.

Listen, we have no options here. Calcium and exercise are our two major weapons in the battle against osteoporosis. If we build muscle mass, strengthen our bones, and add balance and posture correction exercises to our workouts, we can stand tall and avoid that monkey on our backs—a dowager hump.

Physical activity not only will improve our bodies but may improve our psyches. Psychiatrist John Docherty, director of the Center for Innovation in Behavioral Health at New York Presbyterian Hospital/Cornell Medical Center, was quoted as follows in the November 17, 1998, *Washington Post*'s health section: "We know exercise helps regulate biorhythms, which improves sleep, and it enhances energy level and vigor. Exercise is also very important in maintaining physical health and controlling weight, which impacts on self-esteem."

The *Washington Post* article went on to report that in 1996 the U.S. Surgeon General's Report on Physical Activity and Health said, "In general, persons who are inactive are twice as likely to have symptoms of depression than are more active persons." The exercise-mood connection seemed strong enough to bring psychiatrists and psychologists together with exercise specialists to explore "sweat therapy" as an addition to standard treatments of depression.

Working out has lifted my spirits, my mood, and my attitude—and, it is hoped, my butt. Some would say that a feeling of euphoria comes from releasing all those endorphins; I've always suspected it's relief that those thirty minutes of huffing and puffing are finally over.

Some Suggestions for Later-in-Life Beginners

1. Alone is good, but starting your exercise plan with a buddy is better.
2. Review a perspective health club's hours, cancellation procedures, equipment, and trainers.
3. Choose a nationally certified instructor.
4. Get a health screening before starting.
5. Set realistic goals.
6. Exercise in moderation, working at a slow pace toward your goals.

Whenever I'm feeling stressed, angry, or frustrated, or suffering from writer's block, I know my mind-body connection is telling me it's time to spend another thirty to forty minutes stretching, bending, lifting, and flexing.

In addition to the usual run-of-the-mill workouts, my research has turned up a few intriguing and effective alternatives. Body building, yoga, ice dancing, dancing at home to Fred Astaire tapes, playing games rather than working out are among the many choices for staying fit and foxy forever.

And as at any smorgasbord, you can select what appeals to you, ignore what you don't like, mix and match the offerings, and arrange them in a manner to satisfy your unique taste.

If you think you're too old to begin a serious workout, forget about that excuse and get with the program. On Washington's *Fox News at Noon* on January 5, 1999, jazzercise maven Robin Rizzo said, "It's never too late to exercise."

Many of us have said that we're too busy to schedule exercise in our hectic lifestyles. I was guilty as charged. Still plotting the second book in my murder mystery series, I moved from Florida and, once in Washington, contracted to write *Foxy Forever*. While looking for my own apartment, I was staying with my niece. "Good God!" I told her. "I'm too old to be this busy." I was thinking: Be careful what you pray for! My prayers had just been answered, but by responding to an old pattern of behavior, I was wallowing in worry rather than celebrating my better-late-than-never success. And I certainly believed I was far too busy to schedule exercise. Thirty minutes four times a week seemed daunting.

In Florida I threw on a bathing suit, hopped on the elevator, and jumped into the pool in a matter of minutes. As a work-at-home writer in the sunny South, I could exercise while enjoying the company of three other Wonderful Older Women on a daily basis. Our morning pool exercises included stretches, dancing, and aerobics, and we all started our day with great attitudes and lots of energy. Now I was living in Washington, D.C., loving the city lifestyle but missing both the heated pool and the warm bodies who had shared it and helped motivate me to jump higher.

And I was really busy! How could I ever find the time to exercise? Born lazy (sloth has always been my serious sin of choice), I clung to that busy line of dead reckoning like a drowning woman would cling to a life preserver—until my chinos "shrunk in the wash."

I headed for the basement where we co-op owners have our very own gym. Not high-tech equipment but more than satisfactory. Thirty minutes of aerobic exercise combined with weights four times a week. In less than six weeks the chinos fit. But I felt lonely lifting those weights and wanted the company of other women while exercising, so I joined Jazzercise. Guess what? With some judicious time management, I found more than enough hours to juggle the gym workouts and the dance/exercise classes.

Most of you, especially the boomers, do exercise, but even if you have a workout regimen that you love, the following suggestions may inspire or intrigue you to change your routine. Exercise, like food or love, can be in danger of becoming stale or boring.

WOW Workouts

FOXY FOREVER STARS' WORKOUT VIDEOS

These videos can be your primary exercise or used in combination with walking, jogging, or any other outdoor activity. Sometimes exercising only at home alone is too confining. All of these celebrities are over fifty, and all the videos are fun.

Ali MacGraw's Yoga Mind and Body has as its setting the spectacular white sands and deep blue sky of New Mexico. The actress, wearing white leotard and tights, is lithe and limber, and looks lovely. And that's no stretch. MacGraw recommends the stress-reducing yoga movements for mind as well as body.

Joan Collins: Personal Workout is a healthy mix of warm-up stretches; waist, abdominal, and leg exercises; and weight lifting. The scenery is a Barbados beach. Joan's personal trainer is her costar, and they perform an easy routine. Do you know how old this woman is? Saying *ciao* to her sixties, that's how old! And despite the wig, held in place with a turban-like head wrap, she's sexy, Alexis-glamorous, and in sensational shape. Her exercises are sensible and safe. You should be able to breeze through this video the first time.

Mary Tyler Moore's Everywoman's Aerobic Workout combines tummy toners with low-impact aerobics, well performed by a fitness trainer. Moore is now in her sixties, as slim as a girl and as graceful in movement as Laura Petrie and Mary Richards ever were in prime time. I've always known that Mary would turn into a WOW!

My old acquaintance Jane Fonda has a variety of videos on the market. On occasion I still work out to her very first, but any one of them is a fine choice. And Debbie Reynolds's workout routines are like the unsinkable Debbie: zesty and full of life.

For Wonderful Older Women over sixty: Several seniors sang the praises of a video called *Tai Chi for Seniors*, saying its gentle, fluid movements helped relieve their arthritis symptoms, headaches, and stress. The women also felt that these exercises increased strength and infused self-confidence.

Weight Lifting

When are we too old to start pumping iron? Morjorie Newlin's answer would be *never*. The seventy-eight-year-old bodybuilder, who has been turning up on television's morning shows and in the Sunday newspapers' magazine sections, started lifting weights at seventy-two. And this WOW won her first body-building contest that same year.

Weight lifting is a wonderful way to improve your overall health no matter how old you are. People in their eighties and nineties can strengthen their muscles and feel great doing so. In a USDA study at Tufts University, some elderly participants gave up their canes and walkers after they started weight training.

So Newlin, a relative youngster in the weight-lifting game, became my inspiration to really start working on my upper arms. My intentions were good, but then the road to eternally floppy upper arms is paved with good intentions. I confess that I find lifting free weights boring, and while "no pain, no gain" may sound catchy, hoisting those dumbbells can hurt like hell. As a proponent of instant gratification—how long do we have here, anyway?—I'm pushing myself to shape up in record time.

Shortly after I joined the gym, which is located in the co-op's basement, the management arranged for us members, at no extra cost, to spend three hours with a personal trainer, who taught us how to use the equipment and the free weights. The trainer's skillful instructions changed my attitude, if not my ability, about working out with weights.

Variety turned out to be the spice of exercise. I warm up for about three minutes and then combine a seven-minute free-weight session with another ten on the machines; this is followed by ten more minutes doing floor work, yoga stretches, and a cool-down. There you go! Thirty minutes four times a week. Though assured I'll gradually increase my time using free weights and the machines, spending a total of forty or more minutes exercising, I've remained in a happy holding pattern. Maybe I'll think about that tomorrow.

Weighing In with Tips on Weight Training

- Check with your doctor.
- Drink water before, during, and when finished training.
- Don't exercise after eating a big meal; conversely, don't exercise on a totally empty stomach.
- Start slowly; warm up with stretches or on a treadmill. And don't forget your cool-down.
- Have a fitness trainer show you the correct form. Use two-pound weights, and then gradually increase weights as your arms get stronger. After two weeks you should be up to a heavy enough weight that when you lift it twelve to fifteen times, you feel resistance and muscle fatigue.
- Ask a friend to be your spotter when you're working with dumbbells; she can help align you or lift the weight. You can return the favor, and the commitment to working out with a friend increases your show rate.
- Just keep going. Major health risks accompany muscle weakness. You'll be amazed at the improvement in muscle tone that you'll see and feel—and sooner rather than later.
- Weight training is but one aspect of any well-rounded exercise program. Aerobics, flexibility, and balance training are needed as well.

A JUMP START TO CASUAL RATHER THAN ORGANIZED EXERCISING

One of the Wonderful Older Women I interviewed said, "We should stop worrying about our workouts. We should just go out and have some fun." This was one wise WOW. Don't sweat not working up a sweat. When we were kids, we hopped, skipped, and jumped our way through an entire afternoon . . . playing. If we derive pleasure from any physical activity, it becomes fun rather than a *work*out.

As kids we went roller skating, ice skating, bike riding, and swimming. We jumped rope, shot baskets, and practiced ballet leaps. We didn't structure or sign in for exercise time. Instead, we played tag, ran relay races, climbed monkey bars, and reached for the sky while sitting on a swing.

Some of us Wonderful Older Women are revisiting these childhood pleasures and recapturing their health benefits.

Jumping for Joy

As a pigtailed kid I jumped rope while saying "A, my name is Alice," going through the alphabet to "Z, my name is Zelda." But if I stepped on the rope, I lost my turn. Sometimes I'd get all the way to "U, my name is Ursula," but my friend Mary Kay would win the round by jumping without a misstep straight through to Z. We didn't know we were building up our hearts and lungs, strengthening our flexibility, and improving our balance and circulation while burning calories. We were engaged in a game. Jumping has enjoyed a renaissance, and it still provides all those health benefits as well as being one of the least expensive ways to exercise. The only equipment needed is a piece of rope. And jumping's fun factor hasn't changed in the forty or fifty years since our last leap.

You can jump rope in the privacy of your home or backyard as you once did, using a piece of your mother's clothesline, or you can incorporate jumping into your current gym program, or you can select an exercise video that features a rope routine. Jumping rope burns 10 to 12 calories a minute. Muscle tone can be achieved by using the rope as resistance, and when you become a high jumper, you can move to a weighted rope. With practice, a WOW can jump from A to Z with ease.

An Old-Fashioned Walk

If you live less than a half-mile away from the store, *walk*, don't drive—except in the rain, sleet, or snow. You're not the mail carrier. But when the weather is nice, hit the road on foot. I schedule a pit stop at Starbucks for coffee and a chocolate graham cracker—as good as the ones from my high school cafeteria, which had held the chocolate graham cracker good taste record for all those intervening decades until I stumbled into Starbucks. I count on my round-trip journey to use up the calories. Walking is another casual type of exercise; no huffing or puffing, just breathing fresh air and increasing the flexibility of the joints of the lower body.

Most people over fifty have some degree of arthritis. Walking, swimming, and stretching build stronger muscles and bones while reducing arthritic joint pain and stiffness. And like "real" exercise, walking is good for our hearts.

While I walk alone, I often run into a neighbor and am delighted to have a chance to chat and to exchange ideas over a cup of coffee. Exercise is a mind-body connection. If the routine is pleasurable, we are programmed to repeat it.

If you have access to a pool, walking in water is a marvelous way to improve your overall health. If I weren't so intrinsically lazy and if I didn't have to take a bus to get to one, I'd jump right back in the pool.

ICE DANCING AND SUNDRY OTHER SPORTS AND GAMES

The over-sixty set has taken to the ice rink, golf links, tennis courts, dance floors, and other fields of previously unfulfilled dreams with the passion of youth. Peeling many a couch potato off her perch, these activities provide plenty of exercise in the guise of fun and are great social contacts. I met a sixty-something couple who had met and married on the ice.

So pick your passion, or at least a possible interest, and play that sport or game as if your life depended on it. It well may.

YOGA REVISITED: POSITION IS EVERYTHING

Almost twenty-five years ago I lectured on posture, "Walking in Beauty," and taught yoga classes in the grand ballroom during four crossings aboard the *QE II*. I traveled first class in a beautiful cabin, with a guest of my choice invited along to share the voyage. And I found myself listed in the daily program of ship's activities between Joyce Brothers and Lillian Gish. Pretty good billing.

In the early seventies I taught yoga along with a myriad of other self-improvement classes. A colleague who had just returned from teaching yoga aboard the *QE II* while the ship's staff instructor was on holiday called me. Her opening line caught my full attention: "Do you have a passport?" The *Queen Elizabeth* required another substitute instructor. Within two weeks, clutching my passport in one hand and a yoga manual in the other to remain at least a page ahead of the passengers, I embarked on the adventure of a lifetime.

Fortunately, on that first crossing I must have been better prepared than I'd thought. The classes, running every afternoon from four to five, were full. Over two hundred men and women lay supine on the floor of the grand ballroom as I led the opening meditation on that first afternoon. And they kept coming back, packing the ballroom from port to starboard for the five days we were at sea.

On the return voyage I delivered my lecture, worrying about what I could teach these well-heeled, upper-crust, first-class passengers about anything—never mind a topic as nebulous as "Walking in Beauty." Again, the women loved it, joining me in hands-on and best-foot-forward demonstrations. Expert Lecturers booked me for a second round-trip crossing aboard the *QE II,* as well as a cruise to South America aboard the *Oceanic.*

My yoga positions had become almost picture perfect still-life poses, and I felt in almost perfect harmony, mentally, physically, and spiritually. Later, the demands of a full-time Manhattan career, absolutely necessary to support a divorced woman, would tarnish and erode each of those areas. Today, as a writer working and eating alone in my apartment, I'm slowly trying to regain that feeling of total harmony. The yoga I practiced along with my students on the *QE II* is again center stage.

Merging meditation with breathing and movements, yoga is designed to bring us relaxation and better posture while stretching and toning the body. It is also a super stress reducer that can be tailored to any participant's current state of physical fitness. I've incorporated its stretches, lunges, and poses into my warm-ups and floor work, and have combined basic yoga with my aerobic exercises.

If you've never explored the advantages of yoga, perhaps believing it's too slow moving to be effective exercise, I urge you to revisit the lotus position.

Incidentally, the exercise I enjoyed most while aboard the *QE II* was dancing a waltz with Burgess Meredith.

A Balancing Act

Balance is a skill. Use it or lose it! A January 12, 1999, *New York Times* article stressed the importance of a balance-aiding regimen for older people. John Blievernicht, president of Sports Health C.A.R.E. Inc., a Chicago medical rehabilitation clinic, was quoted as saying, "Like anything else in life, balance is a skill. And like any other skill, you've got to constantly practice it to preserve it."

One of my old pool stretches that I now perform on land is an excellent balance-enhancing exercise. The position is achieved by standing tall, with head up and legs together. Stretch your left arm straight out in front of you. At the same time, lift your right leg and hold it out behind you. Then reverse arms and legs. This exercise is called The Swan because if performed correctly, you should resemble a swan. Yes, it takes practice. You might start this exercise by holding on to a bar or shelf with your extended front hand and keeping your raised back leg close to your straight leg. As your balance skill increases, so will your flexibility.

The Tree position also aids balancing; that's right, you're supposed to look like a tree. Stand tall with feet together. Reach both arms over your head and put your open palms together. Raise your right leg and bend it so that your right foot rests on the inside of your straight left leg's knee. Hold for a count of ten. Reverse legs. Hold for a count of ten. Repeat several times.

Many health clubs now offer classes and props for balance training, but an at-home exercise routine that includes yoga can also provide good balance.

The *Anything Goes* . . . Fred Astaire Sings Cole Porter . . . Lazy Woman's Dance Workout

As Faith Whittlesey said, "Remember, Ginger Rogers did everything Fred Astaire did, but she did it backwards and in high heels."

In *Easter Parade*, Fred Astaire danced on the ceiling. My homemade dance/exercise routine is far less ambitious. Like those who only sing in the shower so no one can hear them, I dance alone so no one can see me.

Agile but totally uncoordinated, I flunked my long-ago tennis lessons.

The instructor finally gave up the racket after the tenth session. And taking money while trying to turn me into a tennis player really did qualify as a con game.

Driving lessons were worse. Twenty-seven lessons. Because I kept failing the road test, I kept my driving instructor on retainer. I passed the written exam with flying colors, but then with the inspector sitting next to me, I would miss a stop sign or make a turn into oncoming traffic. I inevitably finished my road test with him in the driver's seat, literally. I also had trouble telling left from right, wreaking havoc with directions; this condition accelerated after I divorced and removed my wedding ring.

If I have a strong leader, I can be successfully whirled around the dance floor, but forget about my following any intricate steps. And as for rhythm, I have none. In the privacy of my home, however, I'm the ghost of glamorous Ginger Rogers and can perform my dance routine without stepping on anyone's foot—and once again play movie star.

While I love Fred Astaire, especially when he's singing Cole Porter, anything goes on my dance floor—from Chubby Checker to George Gershwin. On a lazy day when I don't want to get dressed to do my thirty minutes in the gym, I dance. Wearing my old socks and tattered rag bags, I twirl, twist, and tango. No, I don't dance on the ceiling, but I do use the back of the couch as a ballet barre and sometimes the dust mop as my partner. Though I seldom sing in the shower and never in public— the nuns allowed me in the choir loft only after I promised to just move my lips—I sing along to the music of the old songs that I love. And I dance with the abandon of youth.

With experts extolling exercise as a possible panacea for everything from the common cold—as reported on *Dateline*'s Healthline on February 5, 1999—to a bad back, weak muscle tone, poor posture, heart disease, obesity, depression, and osteoporosis, not exercising could prove fatal. Exercising for thirty minutes four times a week, plus playing some sort of fun and games of your own choice, is an intrinsic part of the foxy forever formula.

Chapter 8

Life Is Just a Bowl
of Cherries

"Diet" is a four-letter word. Let's talk nutrition here. If we are what we eat—or have eaten through all preceding decades—I'm an ambulatory junk-food trash heap. However, my wicked, immature, indiscriminate taste buds may finally have been hoisted on my own foxy forever formula's petard.

For a woman who has been known to create a meal out of bagels topped with cream cheese and jelly and half a bag of chocolate malt balls, washed down with three cups of tea, and considered it gourmet, nutrition may be an even dirtier word than diet!

My body started objecting to my bizarre dining habits, manifested by gassy, nasty stomach distress whenever I overdosed on such favorites as peach pie and French vanilla ice cream, at about the same time that I started to take a serious look at aging well. I guess there really are no coincidences!

Weight gain was not one of my concerns until I was well past menopause. Then like an avalanche everything fell, seemingly overnight, most of it landing on my hips. A man I was dating at the time actually referred to my hourglass figure. This was said to—and about—a woman who had been enjoying a teenage boy's hips, appetite, and metabolism for decades. I remember thinking, "Good God, now I'll have to eat lots of green vegetables and not just my favorite string bean casserole topped with onion rings and laced with cream of mushroom soup. And I'll have to cut back on fat. Neither my stomach nor my hips can take it." What an ugly twist of fate!

Not wanting Pepcid AC, which I'd been using as an after-dinner mint, to become a permanent part of my unbalanced diet, and determined to eat healthier if it killed me, I set out to find a good nutrition formula. I started reading labels. Many contained horror stories that could rival Stephen King's. Half of my recommended daily allowance of sodium could be found in one cup of chicken broth. I had stopped salting my food years ago, and stopped cooking with it, too. Since my recipe for toasting a bagel or English muffin had never called for salt, avoiding it in food preparation hadn't been much of a problem. Except for the bland taste of an unsalted hard-boiled egg, I never really missed salt. The information on the labels explained why: I'll bet there's more sodium in most canned and frozen foods than in Lot's wife's pillar. Adding salt to any of these foods would be as foolish as bringing coal to Newcastle.

By that time too much salt in anything actually affronted my taste buds, so I began buying low-salt foods, from soup to nuts. Today I prefer an unsalted pretzel, especially the sourdough kind—a snack that's actually good for me: no salt added and low or no fat content.

I've always had good blood pressure—120/80. But for several years now, since cutting back on salt, I have, as my doctor said, "the blood pressure of a teenager": 110/60.

Relatively salt free, I still had to deal with that postmenopausal teenage appetite. Satisfying my kiddy cravings while avoiding incipient hippo hips could require more compromise and commitment than I was capable of making.

Admitting that my intake of fatty foods would have to be severely rationed, I latched on to saving my five-meals-a-day plan but acknowledged that I'd have to change my menus. Accepting and implementing those nutritional changes would prove very difficult.

Cookies have been a lifelong staple in my kitchen. "I'll just switch to the fat-reduced ones," I told my friend Doris, the nurse. I often seek her medical counsel during our frequent ten-cents-a-minute phone calls. A few years ago I tried fat-free muffins; they tasted like spongy cardboard. I remained somewhat skeptical. "Do they make a low-fat chocolate graham cracker that tastes like the real thing?" Her long-distance laughter sent me scurrying to the supermarket to read more labels.

Most of the fat-reduced cookies weighed in with hefty sodium, sugar, and calories per serving counts. If I were to eat them with the gusto of my previous cookie consumption rate, I would end up adding weight. My old family favorite, Social Teas, turned out to be the healthiest cookie choice—if I didn't devour an entire sleeve at a sitting.

I had to find a foxy forever formula for eating well that I could tolerate! There had to be a nutrition plan that would allow me to enjoy more than a few of my favorite things. I kept on trucking. My quest eventually led me back to basics. The following guidelines are the result of that search.

Mother Was Right: Breakfast Is the Most Important Meal of the Day

Most Americans eat three meals a day, but statistics indicate that many of us eat only two, skipping breakfast. Though sometimes restricted by work requirements, I have always preferred to eat five, as an active grazer before the term "grazing" was given recognition. And many nutritionists have suggested that five small meals a day are better for us than three big ones. I suspect, though, that those nutritionists were counting calories and had a different definition of "small" than I did.

Whether we eat three or five meals a day, if we're counting calories, *breakfast* is a slim or would-be-slim WOW's best friend. Since our metabolic rate slows down while we sleep, if we skip breakfast, that snail's pace continues, resulting in fewer calories being burned off until we finally do break our fast. If a diet plan calls for 1,200 calories, a quarter of them should be consumed by noon. Select high-carbohydrate foods— bagels, bread, and fruit. Stay away from fatty foods such as doughnuts, cream cheese, and bacon. A scrambled egg with toast (use jelly, not butter) and tea is fine, and so is a small portion of cereal, orange juice, and a cup of 1% milk. A 300-calorie breakfast could include an English muffin with jelly, a peach, and cafe au lait with low-fat milk. I can live with that.

Health and Longevity Can Be Purchased in the Produce Section: The "Apple a Day + Four Other Fruits and Veggies" Theory

The basic food groups—you know, the menu of good stuff that we're to select from and ingest on a daily basis—has always recommended five or more servings per day of fruits and vegetables. Though I seldom came anywhere near that number, I did swallow one multiple vitamin, another 500 milligrams of vitamin C, and 1,200 milligrams of calcium a day. Looking for health in all the wrong places? Not exactly. Most vitamins deliver strong antioxidants, as promised. And we Wonderful Older Women should be taking a multivitamin and 1,200 milligrams of calcium every day. An orange packs such a powerful punch, however, that the National Cancer Institute has referred to it as a complete package of every class of natural anticancer inhibitor known, including vitamin C.

Go ahead, peel and slice one or two. Make a salad of oranges and strawberries, toss in a honey-flavored dressing, and serve on Bibb lettuce. Add a hard roll and a pat of butter—light, if you like—and a slice of turkey. This is my kind of lunch preparation: *easy*.

It turns out that cancer inhibitors can be found in plenty of fruits and vegetables, especially tomatoes. I love a tomato-and-hard-boiled-egg bagel sandwich for any one of those five mini meals I still favor. But you can get your daily dose of tomatoes in sauce, juice, or soup.

Pasta is a wonderful source of carbohydrates. Incidentally, starchy foods such as pasta, bread, and rice can prevent indigestion by absorbing excess stomach acid, so if you're planning a binge, you should at the very least include one starch.

I've always craved pasta, any shape, size, or color, and cooked any style. For a simple, quick, delicious dinner, top your favorite pasta with marinara sauce and a little provolone cheese, and you're dining on one from column A (fruits and vegetables), one from column B (carbohydrates), and one from column C (protein).

And at snack time an apple a day keeps the doctor away. Yes, that old chestnut. Common knowledge. Common sense. Just as our mothers told us.

Are Americans Suffering from Vitamin Information Overload?

"Antiaging dose"—as opposed to the recommended daily allowance—are the current buzzwords used to target-market vitamin and mineral supplements to the aging boomer generation. Manufacturers of these vitamin pills promote their products as an essential part of the purchaser's overall plan to stave off the aging process—an expensive, time-consuming part. For those eager to remain young, there is an amazingly wide variety of vitamins, minerals, and other nutrients out there. If a person attempted to consume all the available supplements, she wouldn't have time to eat— which is how she could reach her recommended levels, please her taste buds, and enjoy a well-balanced meal.

As recently as ten years ago, vitamin and mineral supplements were not considered necessary for people in good health. Today these supplements are big business. According to the *Nutrition Business Journal*, vitamin supplement sales reached almost $5 million in 1997. But are those supplements any more necessary than they were a decade ago?

"I'm too harried to worry about whether my meals supply my nutritional needs, so I take a bunch of pills that do," one woman told me.

"Like what?" I asked

"A cod liver oil capsule, laced with A and D." I shuddered, remembering my mother forcing cod liver oil drops down my throat over half a century ago. The lady laughed at my reaction. "Yeah, I know, but you can't taste it this way. And I take tons of B_{12}, and God knows what all the rest are. But I feel fantastic, so who cares!"

"Did your doctor recommend these supplements?"

"No. My personal trainer did. He swears by them."

A few years ago an advertising section in *Longevity* hyped the antiaging dose versus the RDA of over twenty different vitamin, mineral, and other nutrient supplements. Herb Boynton, chief executive officer of Nutrition 21, the exclusive distributor of chromium picolinate supplements (among the dietary aids that have been promoted by the "natural" weight-loss industry) said, "Retail sales of chromium picolinate this year will reach roughly $100 million, up from 80 million last year." While chromium doesn't have an RDA, the recommended antiaging dose is 200–400 micrograms. Its benefits *may* help dieters lose weight and lower their cholesterol while maintaining muscle tone.

With each new study touting the benefits of the vitamin du jour, a true believer could spend much time and more money in the pursuit of the "right stuff" to prevent aging, heart disease, colon cancer, or loss of sex drive. Yet there is evidence from an ongoing Harvard study that indicates a multivitamin can reduce the chance of colon cancer in women, and many doctors agree that taking one multivitamin a day is a smart health move.

In addition to the multi, calcium supplements are a must for menopausal woman—especially those not on estrogen. Orange juice plus extra vitamin C tablets are used by many to prevent and help treat the common cold.

But what's too much of a good thing? Some nasty reactions from overdosing may include irritation and nausea from iron taken on an empty stomach to internal bleeding from excesses of vitamin E. And a large number of the in-vogue supplements have no official upper-limit tolerance levels. Check with your doctor before mixing and matching vitamins and minerals or arbitrarily increasing their recommended daily allowance.

Foxy Forever Food: The Right Stuff

Pale as a ghost?   Eat iron. It prevents anemia. Iron is found in red meat—yes, it can be good for you—beans, spinach, broccoli, eggs, and liver.

Skin as parched as the Dead Sea?   Zinc sloughs off dead skin cells. It's found in oysters, crabmeat, turkey, red meat—there it is again—

whole grains, nuts, and beans. And for both dry skin and scaly, peeling lips, moisturize: Drink eight glasses of water a day. But you're doing that already, aren't you?

Swelling or puffiness?   If your face, hands, ankles, or feet are puffy, avoid salt. Canned soups are killers, and so are many frozen dinners. Again, check those labels. If you're bruising too easily, increase your vitamin C intake: citrus fruits (drink that daily glass of orange juice), strawberries, tomatoes, broccoli, and squash.

Waging war on wrinkles?   Vitamin A is a weapon. And since we store A in our bodies, it's better to ingest it through food rather than in high doses of vitamin A tablets that exceed the RDA. A is available in carrots, sweet potatoes, leafy green vegetables, peaches, and apricots.

Is Dieting Always the Answer to a WOW's Weight Management?

The French say that after forty a woman should put her face above her figure. Translated, this means too much dieting to keep as slim as possible can make your features too gaunt.

WHAT'S AN IDEAL WEIGHT ANYWAY?

If beauty is in the eye of the beholder, weight must be in the eye of the bearer. Too many Wonderful Older Women are influenced by the pencil-thin images on the runway rather than the realities of life.

The following weight chart for women offered by the *American Medical Association Family Medical Guide* may surprise you. It certainly surprised me!

Height	Weight
4'10"	100–131
4'11"	101–134
5'0"	103–137

5'1"	105–140
5'2"	108–144
5'3"	111–148
5'4"	114–152
5'5"	117–156
5'6"	120–160
5'7"	123–164
5'8"	126–167
5'9"	129–170
5'10"	132–173

Those of us with small frames will be on the lower end of the weight figure; those of us with big bones and frames will be on the high end. The average American woman is 5'4" and weighs between 128 and 135. I know many Wonderful Older Women who fall well within the guideline's weight ranges and yet are always worrying about their weight or starting a new diet. Why? If this weight/height chart is the acceptable range for the American Medical Association, shouldn't these numbers be accepted by us?

After taking into account your body type (frame and bones), if you discover your weight is more than 10 to 15 percent higher than the outer limits, for your health's sake you should reduce.

One blessing that comes with age—and I promise there is more than one—is knowing when our body doesn't feel right. Even if you're not off the charts, you still may want to lose a few pounds.

If Dieting Is the Decision, What's the Best Option?

Browse the bookstores, and chances are you'll find a how-to-lose-pounds book that suits your taste—from *Dieting with the Duchess*, Fergie's Weight Watchers advice book, to *Dieting for Dummies*. *The Better Sex Diet*, *The Cabbage Soup Diet*, and *The Sugar Busters Diet* share shelf space with the standards, such as the Pritikin and Atkins diet plans. In addition to the Duchess of York, who hawked her book on all the morning talk shows, Suzanne Sommers has also written a book that spells out her diet secrets. And those two ladies were just the tip of the celebrity calorie-counting avalanche. Celebrity sells.

According to a recent government report, 50 million Americans will go on a diet this year. With all those potential book buyers, publishers are eager to serve up any new or different diet. Forty years ago a bestseller, *Drinking Man's Diet*, which recommended martinis and steak but scorned starches, was all the rage; my ex-husband swore by it. Today the *Complete Idiot's Diet* is getting raves. Self-help nonfiction books as well as blockbuster novels often come out with catchy titles. Content in either area may be a whole other story. Yet many of these books inspire their readers and encourage goals. They certainly are a viable support system for those dieting on their own.

SUPPORT GROUPS

For those who'd like some group support on their road to reducing, here's a WOW's Weight Watchers report. Ellen Johnson of the Retin A fair face joined the program and reached her desired goal in less than six months. She said the meal plan was easy to follow as well as easy to prepare— and delicious. And at the weigh-in meetings she welcomed the company and encouragement of her fellow dieters. Ellen's now on maintenance, enjoying more flexibility in her food choices and amounts, but she's still counting calories and seldom cheats.

Her newly narrowed rib cage enhances her clothes. She lost inches in all the right places! Ellen does a daily power walk along the Hudson River and aerobic exercises two to three times a week. The exercises alone didn't do it for her, but since combining her workouts with the Weight Watchers program, she looks amazing—a boomer who is truly better than ever.

Or like Rosie O'Donnell, form your own group. Close friends can cheer each other into smaller sizes.

THE MEDITERRANEAN DIET:
GREAT TASTES FOR A HEALTHY HEART

NBC's *Nightly News* on February 15, 1999, reported the success stories of the participants in the Mediterranean Diet study. There were 70 percent fewer cardiac deaths among the heart patients who were placed on the diet. Researchers noted that the Mediterranean people enjoying their own traditional Greek, Italian, and French cuisine had far fewer heart conditions than Americans. In the medical study of those with heart conditions who ate the same foods, the staggeringly good results led the doctors to conclude that all of us, not just patients with heart problems, would benefit from the diet. The menu is sensational, using pasta, tomato sauce, grape leaves, whole-grain bread, and pine nuts, and the food is prepared in the traditional regional dishes. What a way to diet!

THE LENTEN FAST DIET

I'm writing this on Mardi Gras, Fat Tuesday, known in many parts of the world as Shrove Tuesday, the day before Ash Wednesday—the first day of Lent. In Venice they're celebrating Carnivale. Much of South America is partying; this is the last big feast until Easter. And in New Orleans, in what could be the biggest bash of all, it's Mardi Gras! Eat, drink, and be merry, for tomorrow you fast. For all of Lent! For forty days!

My mother lost between seven and twelve pounds every Lenten season of my childhood. For 320 days each year Mom ate pretty much as she liked, knowing that if she gained back those seven to twelve pounds, she'd have another forty days of Lent to lose the weight. The Church has eased up on the requirements of the Lenten season, but the way things were, the fast worked better than most diets. Two meals were to equal but not exceed the size of the third. Fasting, an adult would eat a small breakfast and a light lunch, then a full dinner. No meat was permitted on any Wednesdays during Lent in addition to the year-round Church rule of meatless Fridays. No eating between meals. None! No snacks! Nothing! Except on Sundays when the fast would be temporally lifted. Kids didn't fast; they gave something up—ice cream, soda, the movies. I always gave up candy, even on Sunday. The adults in my house gave up drinking, even on Sunday. Even on St. Patrick's Day! No cocktail hours during Lent. And Mom walked to Mass every day, including Sunday. And the weight rolled off. By Easter the grown-ups looked as great in their new outfits as the kids did.

A forty-day-a-year diet. It certainly worked for Mom.

George Bernard Shaw once said, "There is no love sincerer than the love of food." I suspect he was right. As a card-carrying WOW, I often practice what I preach, but down deep my own nutrition theory hasn't changed: Always follow fresh fish and steamed veggies with a little hot fudge.

Buttons and Bows

Classic clothes, like classic literature, never go out of style. Aim for a classic closet. Begin by tossing the bows. Replace inexpensive buttons, and consider turning yourself into a tailored woman.

For years I worked in the fashion field, foolishly following fads and desperately wanting to look "in." I never found what I was seeking: a signature style. Then when I turned forty, I had a fashion awakening: Classic clothes never go out of style. More important, classic clothes create an ageless appearance. A well-dressed WOW, wearing a natural fiber in a neutral color with timeless style and tailored lines, will be thought of as an elegant woman of uncertain age and not as an old lady trying to look young.

Be wary of garments tagged 100 percent polyester, especially those bearing any resemblance to flower-bedecked, spread-collar shirts from the seventies, arguably the least fashionable decade of the twentieth century.

Retro styles may be here to stay, and no one loves fashion from the past more than I. A childhood spent in double features, learning costume design from the likes of Edith Head and Adrian, strongly influenced my lifelong love affair with clothes. However, there are pitfalls in revisiting and recycling our fashion history. A thrift shop isn't worth its name if you outfit yourself in a jacket equipped with eighties shoulder pads and emerge from the store looking more like Dan Marino than Linda Evans. And the circa 1986 Christian Lacroix pouf dress deserves a decent burial, not a retro resale. Sometimes I think haute couture took a complete nosedive in the mid-eighties.

I'll always favor fashions from the forties, but I tend to emulate the Kate Hepburn look, opting for man-tailored suits and trousers and those wonderful envelope clutches—which my mother also carried—while passing on the perky little hats, strappy high-heeled sandals, and anklets. Those forties accessories should be worn only by Generation Xers.

Forget About Fads

Much of south Florida is a *Glamour* don't. Talk about tacky. There are exceptions—a well-dressed WOW standing out in the sunshine. But consider the following fashion statements: horizontal stripes (which make most of us look like beach umbrellas), clear plastic shoes and handbags (why would you want the whole world to know what you're carrying?), hula hoop earrings; spandex minis, stiletto heels, and color combinations to rival the floats at Mardi Gras. It seems that everyone has worn all of the above—often at the same time.

When I moved south from Manhattan, I lived and worked in the Greater Fort Lauderdale area for ten years. Any number of administrative assistants I'd known in New York City had more fashion savvy than most of the society matrons I met on the Gold Coast. The latter confused fads with fashion, fads that often amounted to too much. These ladies tended to gild the lily—too late. A fad flies by. When I worked in fashion in New York, we used to say, "If you see it riding around on the subway, it's out of style!" By the time a fad—such as one of those ghastly pouf cocktail dresses—appeared at a Fort Lauderdale beach party, it had gone with the whims of the fashion world's trendsetters.

With leisure clothes considered chic, an older man might show up in one of Las Olas Boulevard's finest restaurants wearing wrinkled shorts and sand in his shoes, while his date, circa twenty years younger, might sport a satin slip dress and rhinestone earrings. This casual and ambiguous approach to clothes eventually proved contagious. When I found myself dressing down for dinner, in baggy cotton pants and a T-shirt, and overdressing for a ball, a red chiffon Grecian gown with red velvet ribbons in my hair, I knew it was time to get out of town.

Class and Style Are Not Mutually Exclusive

A woman can have style but no class. A woman can have class but no style.

A rugged individualist can ignore fashion. For the rest of us, following the foxy forever fashion formula will result in putting taste before trends and dressing rich—looking current and classic—even on a fixed income.

How to Have Style and Class on a Budget and Never Pay Full Retail Price

Think Talbots. Today it's not just for the tailored, tweedy set or the fashion equivalent of your mother's Oldsmobile. It's timeless. While some of their clothes are bland—okay, boring—if you stick to the staples, such as well-cut blazers, flattering pleated pants, and oxford shirts in neutral colors, you can build a WOW wardrobe. I have never paid full price at Talbots. Since their classic clothes never really change, each of their end-of-the-season sales affords you a great opportunity to outfit yourself for the following year. At a Talbots outlet in Virginia I actually bought a navy blue linen blazer for twenty dollars and smartly cut sandy beige linen jeans for nine dollars. That jacket and those jeans are my two favorite spring mix-and-match separates. Adding a beige long-sleeved T-shirt, navy and sandy beige scarf, beige loafers, and handbag, I wear them everywhere—from the grocery store to an elegant restaurant.

My niece and I plan two pilgrimages a year, in January and June, to the Talbots outlet to replenish our wardrobes. Their clothes wear like iron, but spots happen. If you have an outlet within a day's driving distance, it's a don't-miss shopping trip.

If you like to shop by catalog, start reading the Lands' End publication from cover to cover. The prices are right, and the clothes probably will outlast your lifetime. Yes, they are plain, not fancy. That's the idea. Once you've developed an eye for putting together a classic closet, you'll see how Lands' End's simple styling can make a fashion statement. And there's an overstock sale section.

Talbots has a catalog, too, but ordering clothes at full price is no bargain. If money is no object, however, head out to Ralph Lauren's Polo, Brooks Brothers, or Burberry. Polo's Madison Avenue flagship store on Madison Avenue and Seventy-second street is housed in an old mansion and definitely worth seeing. Treat these excursions like a visit to a museum; look and admire. You will learn what to look for at their outlet stores, usually located in a mall that is a long drive from wherever I happen to be! Or track down Polo at Marshall's. If you can separate the chaff from the wheat or the traditional from the trendy, you can't beat the prices at Marshall's. The Gap's great American style and their casual clothes can span generations. Shop during sales or at their outlets for white cotton shirts and khakis. The Gap's khakis, like their jeans, come in three lengths. Buying short, I save money on alterations. The British Colonial look—*Out of Africa* meets *The English Patient*, a favorite of mine in both home decorating and fashion—can be found at the Banana Republic.

SIMPLE IS SMARTER

In theory I applaud the concept of the wonderful book that celebrates outrageous freedom from fashion and other constraints, *When I Am an Old Woman I Shall Wear Purple* by Sandra Haldeman Marty. In practice, living my real life, I'd rather be basic in beige, saving my outrageousness for my opinions, my passions, and, as an author, my fictional characters.

Begin with the Basics

You don't need a lot of clothes, just the right ones. A WOW closet should include three basic wardrobe items, all with classic lines and all chosen from one of the six basic colors. You'll want a jacket, trousers, and a dress. Choose your basic color: black, brown, navy, gray, beige, or camel.

Then select an accent color. For example, basic black worn with white accessories is sharp and smart. Or your accent color could be a blue that matches your eyes or another one of the basic colors—or even two. Most of my outfits combine varying degrees of beige, brown, and camel.

THE JACKET

A well-cut, classic, lightweight wool jacket should last a lifetime. Other natural fiber choices are raw silk and wool crepe. An excellent fit is essential. This is not an impulse buy; it's an investment that's worth your time and money. Plan accordingly. You should shop at the better outlets, discount stores, and final 75 percent-off sales at department stores like Lord & Taylor's. I've gotten some of my best winter clothes at their "last chance" spring sale. Buy a designer label and don't be afraid to spend some real money.

Look for small shoulder pads, a supple fit (a cotton sweater should slide under the jacket without causing it to appear bulky), and a length long enough to cover your hips. The correct cut should make you look taller and leaner. You should be able to dress your jacket up or down, wearing with equal élan a lacy camisole or a white T-shirt under it.

THE TROUSERS

Most designers, including Jones, Lauren, Tracy, and Klein, have produced pants to complement many of their jackets and blazers. If your jacket comes with matching pants and they fit, grab them. Then you'll have a suit in a basic color that you can wear anywhere—from a job interview to a night at the theater. Selecting the right trousers can be tricky. Don't assume that because you're size 8 on top that you'll be size 8 on the bottom. Life should be so simple. Depending on your shape and the designer's cut, you might be up to two sizes larger on the bottom. And I actually met one WOW who wore a size smaller on the bottom. That's one out of the one hundred I spoke to this past year.

Look for pleats and proportion in your pants. A Hollywood waist-line—high, with an inch or so of fabric showing above the belt plus pleats in front, below the belt—presents a terrific fashion statement as well as a really slimming look. Even if you're overweight, you'll be able to wear a belt and look great with this cut. I only buy trousers tailored in this style. The way they drape is that flattering! They are much like the trousers that Carole Lombard and Katharine Hepburn favored in the late thirties and early forties. Check out their old movies. *Classic clothes, like classic literature or movies, never go out of style!*

Don't wear your pants too short. They should fall to the middle of the heel of the shoe that you wear with them. When you're having your trousers altered, bring those shoes along!

THE DRESS

Select your basic dress in the style that is best suited to your body shape. Most of us have figures that can be described as square, rectangle, triangle, circle, pyramid, or hourglass. The foxy forever formula for measuring how flattering a dress will look when taken off the hanger and put on the body is predicated on matching the right garment to the right shape. The perfect dress should work with your body shape, and it should fit—no gaps at neck or sleeves, no tight puckering across chest or tummy, no bulges at the thighs, and no drooping at the behind.

The length of a dress depends on the wearer's legs. In general, just above or at mid-knee gives a youthful but not a foolish look. No over-fifty WOW would wear a mini. Some dress styles look great with a mid-calf hemline. If it's a fabric that flows, try ankle length, though not for your wardrobe's basic dress.

A basic dress should be basic. The lines should be simple and the neckline plain, and the fit should flatter your figure. My basic black A-line features a jewel neckline to showcase jewelry or a scarf, long sleeves to cover my far-less-than-perfect upper arms, and a hemline that's just above the knee. Buy your basic dress in the same color and, if possible, in the same fabric as your jacket and trousers. Then you can wear the jacket over the dress, creating a monochromatic ensemble that, properly accessorized, can go anywhere. Voila! You now have the beginnings of a basic wardrobe.

These three basic wardrobe pieces work so well for me that I now have two sets. My black jacket and matching little black dress—which I've had for years, but classic clothes never go out of style—have traveled from funerals to fund-raisers. When I wear the jacket and pants, and add a lacy shell, I have a dynamite theater or cocktail suit. My unstructured beige jacket and wide-leg trousers have a thirties look that takes me from book signings to the racetrack and make me feel as if I'm still playing movie star. The beige sheath dress can stand alone at an informal wedding or dinner party and, when combined with the jacket, goes to town on business.

When deciding proportion and length as well as style, be sure to predetermine your correct body shape.

The Square.   This is a boxy-type figure with wide shoulders and hips. An A-line-style dress that skims a square's waist looks good. A sheath— a rather close-fitting dress with a hint of a waistline and flattering to most figures—can work well for a square shape. A tailored coat dress can slim effectively.

The Rectangle.   If you've been told you have the figure of a teenage boy, you're probably a rectangle. Lean, sometimes lanky, with a small bust and narrow hips, a rectangle is straight up and down. With no visible bumps, you can wear knits—which most women over twenty-one can't dream of doing—and other clinging fabrics. A sheath, A-line, or shift can cover you in style, and a large bib collar will flatter the face and bust-line.

The Triangle.   With broad shoulders, a big bust, and small hips, a triangle should think about a wedge-shaped dress, which is cut wide on top and narrow on the bottom. A tunic with a straight skirt works, too. And a coat dress can minimize a large bust. For evening wear, look for the soft lines of a sheath.

The Circle.   A large, round midsection separates small shoulders from small hips. A portrait neckline or a broad lapel are great looks that will help balance a circle's middle. Shoulder pads are a fashion plus. A circle should shop for relaxed sheaths and styles cut on the bias.

The Pyramid.   Narrow shoulders and a small bust top big hips. Add width to the bust to balance the hips. An empire style or a shirtwaist accentuate a pyramid's waistline. A draped neck or wide collar can enhance the bustline.

The Hourglass. A small waist nestles between well proportioned bust and hips. Tough, huh? An hourglass figure looks great in a wrap dress, a sheath, or a shirtwaist with a wide belt to show off that tiny waist.

ACCESSORIES

"Put your money on your feet!" A fashion maven taught me that years ago. "If a woman's shoes, handbag, and belt are made from fine leathers and classic designs, she can jump into an inexpensive cotton shift, zip it up, and leave the house looking like a million dollars."

To maximize the number of times you wear those three essential wardrobe accessories, and to create a monochromatic head-to-toe look, buy shoes, bag, and belt in the same color as your three basic wardrobe pieces. My stacked-heel, black leather pumps that I can wear with my trousers are three years old; however, they do sport new soles and heels. My "good" little black bag is two years old and beginning to look its age. When I go to New York's Carnegie Hill on my annual summer visit, I head downtown to the August super sale at Crouch & Fitzgerald's Fifth Avenue store to purchase its replacement. I accent my Hollywood waist trousers with my narrow black belt. My two-inch-wide black belt with a gold tone buckle—worn with my three pieces of gold jewelry: earrings, chain, and bracelet—is the only accessory on my basic black dress. Since I'm small, I tend to scale down when accessorizing, but a larger WOW looks wonderful wearing a big, important brooch on a basic dress. Madeleine Albright's strategically positioned pins are her fashion signature.

Black and White and Red All Over

"I'd love to wear black, it's so slimming, but the color makes me look ten years older." At a fashion seminar led by my friend and colleague Diane Dowling Dufour, an expert on "dressing slim" fashions, we heard many variations of that wardrobe worry. Diane suggested two solutions. "Buy black but use white as your accent color and put it next to your face. There's nothing crisper-looking or more dramatic than a black and white color combination. Wear a white blouse, T-shirt, or scarf under your black jacket, tie a white cotton sweater around the shoulders of your basic black dress, or place three strands of pearls on its jewel neckline." Diane demonstrated on a volunteer, draping a white scarf becomingly across the top of a slimming black A-line sheath. Our "model" looked ten pounds lighter, while her face looked ten years brighter. A real scarf trick.

"The other suggestion," Diane offered, "is to opt for a dress in a deep, rich tone such as garnet, forest green, or plum—dark enough to slim down your figure but with enough color to keep your face alive."

I have a third suggestion. Red. It's sensational with basic black, and the right shade of red will flatter any face. That's why we wear lipstick! So pick your accent color from tomato to coral to scarlet, then buy a scarf or blouse and tuck it under your chin. Though I'm a basic-in-beige type of woman, the frames of my Ben Franklin reading glasses are bright red.

A splash of red looks smart, but don't drown yourself in it. Red shoes and a matching handbag are not only not basic, they're downright dowdy. My chiffon evening gown and matching scarlet hair ribbons were prime examples of red gone awry. I'd like to blame it on the Florida heat, but sometimes I do slip and commit a major fashion faux pas, and I alone must accept full responsibility for looking foolish.

Chic mavericks know that fashion rules are made to be broken, but breaker beware. One old guideline that I always adhere to: Shoes should never be a lighter color than your skirt or trousers. Think about it before you scoff. Picture a woman wearing a navy and yellow outfit. It could be really smart. Her buttercup yellow sweater is worn with a navy blue cardigan casually thrown over her shoulders; her straight, slim, well-cut navy skirt, in perfect proportion to her height, ends at her knees; and her panty hose are navy, too. However, our heroine has decided to wear yellow shoes—the exact shade of her sweater—and carry a matching yellow handbag. Her misguided color-coordinated accessories have changed her outfit from terrific to tacky.

Marilyn Monroe has been credited with saying "I wear beige because

I like to be blond all over." That may be the smartest fashion advice I've ever heard. As a blonde—though ash, not platinum—I often opt to be covered in head-to-toe beige. Yes, including my underwear. And when the shoes I'm wearing are of a different color, they're taupe, a darker tone of beige.

WOW Wardrobe Winners: How to Look Like Old Money Rather than Nouveau Riche

To create an ageless look, a WOW needs to coordinate an ageless wardrobe. Most Wonderful Older Women are dressing younger, and we should; however, we don't want to dress like our daughters. Use your three basic wardrobe pieces as a foundation for a chic and classic closet.

Fashion filters down from the runway to reality. From films to fairgrounds. From *People* to people. The rich and famous can have really bad taste, and their flamboyance, their fat lips filled with collagen, and their trashy trends can sweep across the country. Don't get caught up in the maelstrom. Instead, seek a fashion role model and follow her lead. Look at the Ralph Lauren ads; his models are the prototypes for that old money look. Check out Carmen!

Carmen, whose modeling career spans over fifty years, is my fashion role model. Of course, since she's tall and I'm short, I adjust accordingly. In a *McCall's* fashion layout a few years ago, Carmen wore classic styles in neutral colors, accented with a splash of color, with the élan of an ageless woman. Her smartly shaped just-above-the-shoulder-length gray hair looked great, almost matching a monochromatic off-white (with just a tinge of gray) turtleneck sweater featuring dolman sleeves; this topped softly pleated pants and flat tobacco-colored loafers. I ran out and bought Liz Claiborne's version of Carmen's look. Since I'm too small for dolman sleeves and a turtleneck is not my favorite style, I bought a jewel neck-lined long-sleeved sweater and matching front-pleated wool pants. And my off-white had a hint of beige rather than gray, which is better for my skin tone and hair color.

CAN A CLASSIC CLOSET CONTAIN CLOTHES OF MANY COLORS?

Yes! Just don't wear them all at the same time. One reason that I buy so many monochromatic outfits is that I love neutral tones. Another is that I'm short, and a long unbroken vertical line in the same shade makes me look taller. A red blouse, white belt, and blue skirt, for example, would break that line and make me appear shorter and wider, albeit patriotic.

As we age, bright colors are flattering, especially when worn near the face, so why wouldn't we want to wear them? Think of the neutral tones as your base; then, like an artist, start adding splashes and dashes of the colors you love and that look great on you.

Scarves in jewel tones—ruby red, aquamarine, emerald, sapphire, turquoise, depending on your skin tone—will warm and flatter any face. A dress or suit in your favorite hue, whether it's coral, peacock blue, or a flattering pastel, worn with neutral accessories will look wonderful. If you have a good figure and tomato red is your color, wear a sheath in that shade, and *wow* the room. But I wouldn't suggest a coral blouse with a bright blue suit, worn with matching blue shoes and topped off with a multicolor plaid scarf. Or a red coat worn over a purple dress. That's why a coat—unless you own four or five of them—should be in a basic color. You can throw black or camel over almost anything.

When Cokie Roberts, *This Week*'s cohost, veers from basic neutral colors and puts on pastel, such as a pale blue suit, she opts for a matching pale blue blouse. Cokie's color-coordinated chic is a look I try to emulate. Diane Sawyer, another of TV's best-dressed anchors, almost always wears neutral monochromatic colors in basic styles and always appears classy and classic—a real WOW.

Underneath It All Lays the Foundation

Wearing the wrong underwear can ruin a good day. Being foxy forever doesn't mean we have to sacrifice comfort for chic. As a teenager in the fifties I wore a panty girdle under all my knit or sheath dresses. God knows why, since I had neither hips nor stomach to constrain. And I

The Foxy Forever Foundation Formula: Easy Essentials

- Smooth, no-lines sweater bras to wear under knits. They can be lightly padded. Or try a Bali underwire to structure a fuller bust.
- French-cut Jockey for Her underpants. These have a comfortable natural waistline but no panty line.
- Control-top hose to keep tummy smooth and flat. The correct size should be comfortable.
- When relaxing, wear your old, comfortable underwear. But when you're all dressed up and have somewhere to go, don't leave home without your own Wonder Bra.

layered three petticoats plus a small hoop (as decreed by that decade's disastrous designs) under my mid-calf full skirts. I could barely navigate through the subway doors.

As a WOW I have taken a vow never to wear an uncomfortable piece of underwear. I couldn't believe that in the last days of the twentieth century trendy teens—as well as should-be-smarter-than-slaves-to-fashion older women—were duped into wearing bustiers. They reminded me of the torturous merry widow, a long-line killer bra from my bridled youth.

How to Select a Swimsuit Without Becoming Suicidal

As far as I can tell, there isn't any way. If you discover one, write to me at St. Martin's Press. In the meantime, bring along your dearest, closest, most trusted friend who is at least as old as you are. Pick out the six best possibilities together, go to the dressing room, put on a blindfold, try those suckers on, and let her choose.

Anything Goes

Well, of course it does. Hasn't it always? Not all of us are cut from the same pattern, and a WOW who marches on another runway can create her own foxy forever fashion formula—or ignore fashion altogether. As for me, after a lifelong love affair with clothes, I enjoy sharing my acquired knowledge and my appreciation for classic style. I also accept, however, that part of the fun of fashion is that all its formulas are variable.

Moonlight Becomes You

It's the daylight that drives us to cosmetic surgery! Is there a woman approaching fifty who hasn't considered some sort of plastic surgery? I may know of one—at least that's what she says. But thinking about a face-lift or a tummy tuck is a long way from being wheeled into the operating room. The procedure that will firm a jaw and tighten jowls calls for a scalpel, not a magic wand. It's *surgery*! And our health plans won't cover the costs. Determined-to-look-better Wonderful Older Women have found ways to pay the price. But even with all the hype promoting nips and tucks, many more Wonderful Older Women have decided to keep the face they have, despite its wrinkles and sags.

Shortly after turning fifty, author Sue Hubbell removed the mirror from her bathroom and found a "better self-image." Not seeing a reflection of my creased and puffy morning face no doubt would enhance my own inner feelings of self-worth, but then I wouldn't be able to improve on my outer image.

Regarding cosmetic surgery, my stand remains firmly pro-choice.

What Is a Face-Lift, and What Results Can We Expect from One?

I met with two reputable plastic surgeons and had long interviews with several women in various stages of preparing for or recovering from rhytidectomy, the medical term for a face-lift. All the questions you've ever had about a face-lift, but didn't want to pay the plastic surgeon's consultation fee to ask, were answered.

THE CANDIDATE

If your jowls, jawline, and neck are sagging but your skin still retains some elasticity, you're a perfect candidate for a face-lift. Basic good bone structure can also help achieve great results. Most patients are in their forties to their sixties, but women and men well into their seventies and eighties have had wonderful results. Be realistic. While a lift usually boosts your spirits along with your sagging skin, it can't raise your health or energy level. Don't expect to look decades younger; do expect to look fresh and firm. And be prepared for compliments.

"Everyone says I look great," Bonnie P. told me three weeks after her surgery. "Most people ask, 'Did you have your hair cut or what? You look so different.' Only one guessed that I'd had a face-lift. But I'm so thrilled with the results that I'm telling everyone!"

THE OPERATION

A face-lift procedure removes excess fat, tightens muscles, and redrapes the skin on the face and neck. Bonnie's jowls were history, and her jawline appeared minus-fifteen-years firmer. I'd known Bonnie for several years prior to her surgery, and as her pre- and post-op pictures confirmed, there was a dramatic difference in her before and after face. You can opt for a face-lift alone or combine it with other procedures such as eyelid surgery or a forehead lift.

The operation takes about four hours but can run longer if you're having your lids or forehead done. The length of the procedure and where the incisions are made depend on your facial structure and your surgeon's skill. You really want to shop around for a first-class plastic surgeon!

In general, an incision starts at the temple, above the hairline, goes down the front of your ear, and then behind the earlobe to the lower scalp. A small incision is made under the chin in order to work on a sagging or wrinkled neck.

The facial skin is separated from the fat and muscle below it. To contour the chin, fat is trimmed or suctioned from the neck and chin. The surgeon tightens the underlying muscles and tissues, then redrapes the skin over the face, snipping off the excess. Stitches close the incisions and hold everything together. Sometimes, especially if there is a forehead lift involved, metal clips are used on the scalp.

After the surgery, a tube is usually inserted under the skin behind the ear for the next few days to drain the blood, and the head is loosely wrapped in bandages to reduce swelling and bruising.

The following is my own informed and considered opinion: Do not have a face-lift performed as an outpatient. Choose a doctor who will put you in a hospital and keep you there overnight. Many doctors opt to operate in an office-based facility, an outpatient surgery center, or even in a hotel room, and send their patients home the same day. A face-lift is major surgery, with all the potential red flags of any serious procedure, and you should spend at least twenty-four hours recovering in a hospital where you will be monitored and where emergency treatment is available if needed.

THE RECOVERY

It is not as it was in the old movies where the doctor removes the patient's bandages, hands her a mirror, and a brand-new beautiful face is unveiled. In real life when the bandages come off—from one to five days after surgery—the patient looks as if she took a direct hit from a truck.

Over a dozen years ago I had a face-lift. With the bandages on, I looked like *The Mummy*; when the bandages came off, I looked like a very black-and-blue *Frankenstein* monster. Talk about a fat head! And it took almost three weeks for the discoloration to go away. The swelling took much longer. By the end of a week, swathed in scarves that covered my white gauze helmet and wearing big Jackie O sunglasses that hid the black stitches sewn around my eyes, I felt well enough—though I certainly didn't look it—to venture out to lunch at a friend's house.

In the ensuing years there has been a great deal of medical progress, and recovery has become much speedier. Most patients are up and about in a day or two, but doctors still advise taking it easy for the first week of recovery. Your face will be tender, you should treat your skin and hair with gentleness, and you need to remember that you have just gone through major surgery. Doctors advise getting plenty of rest; allow your face time to heal and your body to regain its energy. Don't partake in exercise, heavy housework, or sex for at least two weeks. You can walk and stretch. Stay away from alcohol, steam baths, and saunas. And avoid exposure to the sun for several months. Based on my own experience, I'd say forever!

The women I interviewed seemed to have experienced far less trauma than I had, although they all agreed that they had been shocked by their bruised, puffy faces when their bandages were removed. And as I had done, they all complained of numbness, a normal side effect that disappears in time.

If ongoing pain or sudden swelling occurs during the recovery period, call the doctor. There shouldn't be much real pain after the operation, though there is plenty of discomfort. My head felt like a ten-ton balloon for the first few days. And I couldn't chew. I lived on liquids and sipped lots of chocolate milkshakes.

Trauma to my psyche proved to be as bad as my bruises and swollen head. My features looked distorted, my jaw felt stiff, and my scars were raw, ugly, and scary. Every time I caught sight of my fat head in a mirror, I thought, What if my face stays this way? What if God has punished me for my vanity?

It is important even while completely crazed to elevate your head and keep it as still as you can for several days to reduce swelling. I slept with three pillows, almost sitting up. The drain is usually removed two days after surgery, and the stitches come out about four or five days later. In a few weeks, and sometimes sooner, you should be feeling great, and you and your new look will be ready to face the world.

THE RESULTS

I met Lucky S. almost three months after her face-lift. Except for shiny, slightly ruddy skin (it turned out that she'd had a peel several months before her surgery), this fifty-something woman appeared not only healed, healthy, and glowing but to be thirty-something. You would never know she had had a procedure performed recently or ever, her lift looked that natural.

We were in Bonnie's car, driving from Fort Lauderdale to Miami to meet the Costa Rican plastic surgeon who had operated on both women. My friend Diane, curious about the cost of a tummy tuck in Costa Rica, had come along for the ride. Since none of my friends ever lets me drive—yes, I am that bad behind the wheel—I listened to the ladies and took lots of notes.

Both Lucky and Bonnie had done a great deal of research on the pros and cons before flying to Costa Rica for their face-lifts.

"What convinced you?" I asked Lucky.

Seated next to Bonnie in the front seat, Lucky turned to face me. The hot Florida sun cast a halo around her blond hair. "The three R's were my main concerns: repercussion, reputation, and recourse. During my consultation, the doctor addressed each of those questions, completely convincing me that Costa Rica was the place to have my operation and that he should be my plastic surgeon."

"Not to mention," Bonnie added, "that even counting airfare and hotel, it's thousands of dollars cheaper than here in the States."

I felt excited; I would be having my own consultation with Bonnie and Lucky's surgeon that afternoon.

Bonnie had returned home less than two weeks ago after spending ten days recovering from her surgery in Costa Rica. Her new face was less than a month old. She still had some swelling, but the pouches were gone from under her eyes, as were her jowls, and her jaw was firm.

With great delight Bonnie told us, "Someone I met in the supermarket said that I now look like I'm my own daughter."

Knowing that despite the compliments and the thrill of feeling young again, Bonnie harbored some concerns regarding her healing process, I asked, "What about that indentation on the side of your face?"

"That's one of the things I'm going to discuss with the doctor." Bonnie sounded positive. The results of her face-lift seemed to have included a permanent infusion of self-confidence.

Lucky had to love her results. Her face appeared totally unaltered. She'd chosen not to have her eyes done, and I thought the fine lines that formed when she smiled only added to her naturalness. And I wondered, not for the first time, why other women's wrinkles always seemed so much more attractive than my own.

"You could be any plastic surgeon's poster woman, Lucky. Tell me about your three reservations, those three R's."

She smiled. "Well, to start with, I'd be in Costa Rica all alone. My husband thought I was crazy but said if I felt I needed a lift, to go ahead, but he never offered to come with me. I don't speak Spanish. What would I do if something went wrong? Who would even understand that I needed help?"

"The repercussions?" That fear certainly would be one of my major concerns regarding surgery in a strange country.

"Well, as it turned out," Lucky said, "patients stay in the hospital for three days—as opposed to one day in the States—under close monitoring by an English-speaking nurse. They then continue recovering at a nearby hotel for the next week where he visits them every day."

Bonnie jumped in. "You don't have to worry about the doctor's reputation, Noreen. Lucky thoroughly checked out his credentials and even arranged to meet post-op patients in his Miami office. And as you know, I did my homework, too, and investigated four other doctors before selecting this one. He's wonderful!"

"And recourse?" I asked. "What happens if a serious problem should arise after you guys have been home awhile? Would you have to fly back down to Costa Rica for repairs?"

"Like the hole in my head?" Bonnie laughed. "That's one of the reasons he keeps an office in Miami. He can't operate in America, but he can refer you to a local doctor if something needs to be fixed."

I couldn't wait to meet this paragon.

Another friend had her face-lift done locally. Unlike mine, it had included a forehead lift. I visited her in the hospital; she was swathed in bandages, sported metal clips in her head, and was feeling some pain. I remember thinking that she still looked better than I did a week further along in my recovery.

When recovering, she complained of tightness, that her face felt numb, but those feelings passed in about six weeks.

Of course, the local lift had cost much more than Bonnie's Central American adventure.

My own face-lift, then almost eleven years old, had started to droop. For the last decade I had looked more than a decade younger than I was.

No more. My lift had definitely dropped, my jawline had softened, and my neck looked loose. Could I really face another operation? Could I afford one? Could Costa Rica be the answer?

THE DOCTORS

The doctor reminded me of Cesar Romero. Tall, with silver hair and attractive, he oozed Latin charm and fatherly warmth combined with professional concern and medical smarts. He impressed me. I liked him a lot. Even more surprising, considering that his Miami office was a condo apartment, my friend had actually stepped into the bedroom for an examination of her thighs. And his office manager/sales representative turned out to be a travel agent.

The entire visit and consultation felt like a mini trip through the *Twilight Zone*. However, the doctor's manner, professionalism, peer recognition, and surgical skills proved to be impeccable. Several of his post-op patients wandered in. All greeted him with great affection and admiration. And each of their results, for their various stages of recovery, seemed extraordinarily successful.

While we were sitting on the living room couch, he carefully examined my face, taking it into his hand and turning it this way and that, first toward the sunlight and then toward the bright lamp light. "Your eyebrows are perfectly positioned, and your brow is unlined," he said with a slight Spanish accent. "You do not need a forehead lift." Then he admired the work of my surgeon, Dr. Papillon—I'd always found it amusing that my plastic surgeon had a name that translated into "butterfly"—and went on to chat with a post-op woman who almost genuflected as he approached. I went on to his office manager/sales representative/travel agent to discuss the costs.

Gisela Zacapa, who represented Imperial Travel as well as the doctor, was gracious, patient, informative, and could answer all questions while covering all contingences. The face-lift surgery would be part of a package deal, and there were five different package options to choose from depending on the surgical procedure or procedures involved. The letterhead of the information sheet that I reviewed with Gisela featured Imperial Travel's logo, address, and phone number.

Each package's all-inclusive cost included:

round-trip air transportation from Miami to San Jose via Lacsa
   Airlines
transfers from and to the airport, hospital, and hotel
hospitalization expenses (three nights)
first-class hotel (six nights)
doctor's fees

I found it interesting that the surgeon's charge had been relegated to the bottom of the price list.

Stapled to the sheet were three business cards: Gisela's; the doctor's, which included phone numbers for his Miami and Costa Rica offices and his home phone (which really impressed me); and one containing a list of the medical tests to be completed before leaving for Costa Rica.

The last item was a colorful brochure for the Hotel Sangildar proclaiming its amenities "the finest in Costa Rican hospitality." Following their surgeries, Bonnie and Lucky had stayed at this hotel. The doctor visited them every day, as promised, and they both raved about the hotel's service, charm, convenience, and accommodations. And both women assured me that their inability to speak Spanish presented no problem either at the hotel or during their hospital stay.

This consultation took place almost three years ago. My friend's thighs and trip would have cost $1,900. My all-expenses-included Costa Rican face-lift would have been under $4,000. For different reasons, neither of us had cosmetic work in Costa Rica; however, I remain very impressed with the doctor and his results.

Last year, choosing a surgeon with great care, I went for another consultation.

During my residency in south Florida I had come in close contact with hundreds of face-lifts. And that's the problem: If a face-lift is done right, after six months when the swelling is all gone, no one except your hairdresser should be able to guess that you ever had one.

There was one very expensive, stretched-out-to-the-sides lift that many society women were facing the world with. I dubbed it the Palm Beach Puss. As if that scary look, photographed frequently and featured in the *Sun-Sentinel* and *Palm Beach Post* society sections, wasn't bad enough, I also witnessed some tragic results from bargain basement cosmetic surgery.

Beware of surgeons who take out full-page glossy ads in the Sunday papers, promising to carve you into a new woman. Their advertising budget may be much higher than the money they've allocated to ensure the safety of their outpatient operating room procedures.

One WOW had eyelid surgery performed in just such an environment in order to save money, and she wound up suffering from sever financial and physical repercussions.

Anna (not her real name), a very attractive, hardworking single mother who is putting her daughter through college, can't afford to close up her one-woman shop even for a few days. She allowed a plastic surgeon who ran an outpatient cosmetic surgery center to address a gathering of her clients and friends in order to promote his services. In a sort of barter agreement, she would have her upper and lower lids done for free!

Both the surgeon and Anna were happy with their arrangement. She was back at work the day after the surgery, but behind the dark glasses, the results were bad. One eye was askew and appeared sore. The doctor agreed to "fix" the problems at no cost—or, rather, only for the cost of the anesthetist and the operating room. The "fix" didn't work. In a short time, with the same doctor performing a second repair surgery, Anna returned to the operating table. That night, bleeding heavily from one eye, she drove herself to the local hospital's emergency room. She then visited another surgeon. His diagnosis: Too much skin had been removed from her lids, which was why she couldn't shut her eyes. The second doctor performed a skin graft from her fanny to her face. Over a year later, having suffered from days filled with discomfort and wide-awake nights, Anna felt that her eyes didn't look right, and she still couldn't close her right eye. When I last spoke with her, she was considering more corrective surgery.

In the end, though, Anna sued the center. She not only never collected a cent, but she wound up spending over $3,000 to repair their work.

So I sure knew what I didn't want in a plastic surgeon!

I also knew what I did want. For several years I served as vice president of public relations on the board of directors of Fort Lauderdale Sisters Cities International. Dr. Richard Ott, M.D., P.A., attended one of our meetings to promote one of his favorite projects. Interplast South, an all-volunteer organization founded by Dr. Ott, provides reconstructive plastic surgery for children in developing countries. The group has an ongoing relationship with the country of Honduras. In addition to sponsoring the surgeons' trips, Interplast South brings children back to Fort Lauderdale when they require more extensive treatment. The moment I saw the pictures of the miracles this good man had performed on the faces of those children, I knew he had the heart of a humanitarian and the hands of an artist.

A WOW whom I'd never suspected of having a face-lift confided that she'd gone to Dr. Ott several years earlier after "interviewing" several other doctors. Then another friend who was about to turn fifty, and as a birthday present had set a date for Dr. Ott to operate on her, shared the names of two more of his former patients with me.

My about-to-be fifty friend emerged from surgery looking thirty-five and as if a scalpel had never touched her face. A few months later, I sat in Dr. Ott's waiting room.

I brought lots of concerns to the consultation. In addition to drop, I now had lots of lines, especially around the mouth. Ignoring my dermatologist's advice and my own common sense, I had spent far too much time in the sun, trying to tan but too frequently getting burned right through my number 15 sunblock. If I have one piece of painfully acquired wisdom to share, it's this: Only mad dogs and foolish women wanting to scorch their skin go out in the noonday sun.

Dr. Ott was every bit as competent and as personable as I had expected him to be, and his comments and suggestions regarding any future plastic surgery that I might consider were both honest and intriguing.

First, he complimented Dr. Papillon's Canadian handiwork, even calling his nurse in to inspect my face. "This surgery is twelve years old!" Dr. Ott told his nurse. "Just look where her scars are. Aren't they great?" Dr. Ott turned back to me. "This man was using the same surgical technique I use, long before it became popular in the States."

The nurse said, "I thought she looked good for her age, but I never would have guessed she ever had a lift!" I guess that was a compliment to Papillon's skill and, possibly, to me. I gathered that this woman usually could spot a face-lift across a crowded room.

"Well," I explained, "I went to Canada to save money!" Manhattan prices, even back then, were out of sight. I had a wonderful French friend who lived in Plattsburgh, just across the border. Janine hooked me up with the doctor, brought me for my consultation, and then drove me to the hospital on the day of the surgery and home on the day after. She also ferried my mummy-wrapped head and still wobbly body back and forth across the Canadian border for all post-op visits. We were the recipients of some startled stares and puzzled questions from the immigration officers. I've often wondered what they suspected I was smuggling under all that gauze. Janine also put me up in her guest room and played nurse for three weeks.

Dr. Ott recommended a basic face-lift. As the first surgeon had pointed out, no forehead lift was needed. Using his fingers, Dr. Ott pulled up my brow to make his point. The startled expression that stared back at me in my handheld mirror was scary, reminding me of the dreaded Palm Beach Puss. And he wouldn't do my bottom lids again. "There's not enough skin to remove." Thinking of Anna's painful results, I listened with respect to what he said. "The top lid is a little loose, but that's up to you. It doesn't need to be done."

"What about these lines on my cheeks?"

"Pull the sides of your face up gently, like so." Dr. Ott gently raised the loose skin under my cheekbones. "See how those lines have diminished? They seemed to have vanished!"

He was right!

If I ever have the time and the money, maybe one day I will have that chin lift.

Young at Heart

How to keep our hearts young and our livers, spleens, kidneys, and lungs middle-aged. As we age, that old bromide—being beautiful on the inside—takes on a whole new meaning! According to a Mayo Clinic Health Letter report, we're going to live longer than we thought we would. As we enter a new century and a new millennium, life expectancy at birth is over 50 percent higher than it was a century ago—seventy-six years today versus forty-seven years. And one out of every twenty-six boomers is now expected to live to be one hundred. Those statistics will only get better!

What we do with that precious gift of extra time will pretty much depend on how healthy we can keep our vital organs.

Starting at the Top

USE YOUR BRAIN: PLAYING MIND GAMES

Before television created what has been called a nationwide brain drain, people actually had to entertain themselves. Families and friends played games together. Today, if someone is in the middle of a chess game, chances are there is no live opponent, that she or he is all alone, deciding how to play that rook on a computer screen. Interactive games should require other warm bodies to compete with, to try to outsmart, to duly impress—and to gloat over if you win!

Have you ever forgotten the name of a famous Hollywood star from your salad days at the movies? This happened to me about two years ago. And of all the people whose names might have been better forgotten, I drew a blank on Rita Hayworth! When I was about ten and she was *Gilda*, I probably knew as much about Rita and her romances—both on and off the screen—as Louella Parsons and Hedda Hopper. "You know," I sputtered to my young neighbor as if she could fill in the blanks, "the redhead who was married to Artie Shaw and Orson Welles!" Of course, being Generation X, she didn't have a clue.

At two o'clock that morning, Technicolor images of Gene Kelly twirling the *Cover Girl*, while her beautiful hair whirled around behind her, danced through my dreams. I bolted up in bed, wide awake, and shouted, "Rita Hayworth!" If I'd still been playing Trivial Pursuit, as I once had done on a twice-weekly basis, I'm certain I wouldn't have suffered a senior moment that lasted twelve hours.

In Washington my niece, another old film buff, and I watch, review, and rehash videotapes from the golden age of movies as if their stars were still shining over Hollywood. I guess for some of us they will always twinkle. And I have had no lapses in stardust memories since my mind temporally misplaced Rita Hayworth. Now I'm thinking of starting a Trivial Pursuit game in the building. The Silver Screen edition!

I've joined a Scrabble club. I love words, but more important, as a writer, words are my business. The game and I have a long history. When I was a teenager, my mother and I played Scrabble together several nights a week. Decades later I taught my son to play, and eventually, as his grandmother had done before him, he played to win.

Finding new friendly foes to challenge my Scrabble skills has added to both my vocabulary and my social life.

Most Americans watch between thirty and fifty hours of television a week. God knows how many hours they log on their computers. We're working longer and spending less quality time with the people we love. Even the older, pretelevision and former board-game-playing crowd has become hooked on the Internet. Never mind great literature, some of us don't have time for the daily newspaper; reading has taken a backseat to the Movie of the Week. Yet the mind needs stimulation, not a daily dose of pap. Exercise your imagination, your creativity, your betting ability. Poker, gin rummy, bridge, and Bill Clinton's favorite game—well, his favorite card game—hearts are fun and challenging ways to give your brain a workout.

In addition to sharpening her mind, a WOW who plays games will never be lonely. Someone is always looking for a fourth for bridge. And I'll bet that there's a Scrabble player searching for a vowel or a consonant right under your own proboscis.

A SENIOR MOMENT ISN'T THE START OF SENILITY

While I may remember Rita, I sometimes forget why I've gone into the kitchen. As soon as I walk back to the living room, I recall I needed a small trash bag for the bathroom wastebasket—or whatever my mission had been. On a recent Today *Show*'s Forever Young segment, a doctor explaining the early signs of Alzheimer's assured us that we did not need to worry about those senior moments when we've forgotten why we're in front of the refrigerator, but we should start to worry if we've forgotten what the refrigerator is.

YOUR MIND: USE IT, DON'T LOSE IT!

Continue to work on your memory and word power. Interact with real people, not just the computer, and you won't just be improving your brain. According to researchers at the State University of New York at Stony Brook, a fun activity such as dinner with a friend can actually boost our immune systems for up to three days by releasing antibodies that ward off minor illnesses.

If we exercise our brains as well as our bodies and maintain an active social life, we'll retain those precious memories and remain bright, quick, and foxy forever.

You Gotta Have Heart!

A quick quiz to enhance your quality of life and keep your heart throbbing:

1. Is it true or false that heart attack symptoms can be different in women?

2. Which of the following can keep a heart healthy?
   a. reducing stress
   b. adding grains, pasta, and beans to your daily diet
   c. stopping smoking
   d. all of the above

3. Which of the following is not an unsaturated fat?
   a. olive oil
   b. coconut oil
   c. canola oil
   d. safflower oil

4. How many gallons of blood does the heart pump every day?
   a. 100
   b. 500
   c. 1,200
   d. 2,100

5. What does severe narrowing of the arteries result in?
   a. angina
   b. heart attack
   c. stroke
   d. all of the above

6. Is it true or false that palpitations (irregular heartbeats) usually indicate heart trouble?

7. Is it true or false that heart disease is the number one killer of women in the United States?

And the answers are:

1. *True*. Ignoring the symptoms of a heart attack may prove fatal. Almost 50 percent of all heart attack deaths occur within the first hour after the onset of symptoms. George Washington University Hospital's winter 1999 issue of *Health News* reports that women are slower to go to a hospital than men because they don't realize they're having an attack. According to the American Heart Association, these are some of the common warning signs of a heart attack: uncomfortable pressure; fullness or pain in the chest that lasts longer than a minute or goes away and comes back; pain that spreads to the shoulders, neck, or arms; chest discomfort with lightheadedness, fainting, sweating, nausea, or shortness of breath.

Women may also have these less common signs: dizziness or nausea; unusual chest, stomach, or abdominal pain; palpitations, cold sweats, or paleness: difficulty breathing.

If you ever experience any of the above symptoms, get to the hospital immediately. The life you save will be your own.

2. *d, all of the above*. I bet you had this one right! We all know that stress, smoking, and a poor diet are the three major contributors to heart disease, and unlike a family history of heart disease or diabetes, we can eliminate these risk factors. And watch that blood pressure.

3. *b, coconut oil*. Saturated fats wreak havoc with cholesterol. Since high cholesterol is one of the most controllable risk factors, a dietary change can help prevent heart disease. Saturated fats that raise your cholesterol count are found in animal products such as butter, milk, and fatty meats, and in palm or coconut oil. A diet of low-fat dairy products, complex carbohydrates—such as grains, pasta, and beans—and lots of fruits and veggies will lower your cholesterol and reduce your weight.

4. *d, 2,100*. The heart is the strongest muscle in our bodies and the most important! The heart beats about 100,000 times a day, sending 2,100 gallons of blood coursing through our vessels and arteries. When the heart is healthy, blood flows freely through the coronary arteries, and the correct amount of oxygen travels through those arteries back into the heart's muscle—making the heart the only one of the body's muscles to supply its own energy. Awesome, isn't it?

5. *d, all of the above*. Heart disease doesn't develop overnight. A gradual buildup of fatty tissues in the arteries is often caused by ignoring

risk factors such as smoking, high cholesterol, and high blood pressure. The damaged lining then attracts cells carrying cholesterol and other fatty substances, narrowing the arteries and reducing the flow of blood to the heart. Severe narrowing can result in angina or a heart attack—or, if the blockage occurs in the arteries leading to the brain, a stroke.

The National Stroke Association reported that 97 percent of people over the age of fifty who were questioned in a Gallop poll didn't know even one warning sign of a stroke. A stroke is an attack on the brain that requires immediate action. It is the number one cause of disabilities in adults. Its symptoms include numbness, weakness, or paralysis of an arm or leg, blurred or decreased vision, difficulty in speaking, and loss of balance. Most strokes are preventable, but we should determine our risk factor. We can educate ourselves on both prevention and treatment by talking to our doctors or calling the National Stroke Association.

6. *False.* We all occasionally experience irregular heartbeats. There is no such thing as a "normal" rhythm. When a heart skips a beat, the jump is called a palpitation. It can be scary, but most of the time—unless accompanied by other symptoms—it is harmless. Stress, stimulants, and lack of sleep can make a heart jump. Reactions to the overuse of laxatives or diuretics cause irregular heartbeats. If palpitations accompanied by dizziness occur more than once in a month or persist for a month or longer, see a doctor.

7. *True.* Coronary disease kills over 360,000 women a year. So treat your heart with respect and tender, loving care.

Cancer Prevention

If cancer tends to be lurking in your family tree, you should be taking aggressive action, learning all you can about preventive strategies, having more frequent checkups, and taking appropriate screening tests on an annual basis.

BREAST CANCER

You could be at risk if you have a family history (mother or sister), if you menstruated before ten or had your first child after thirty, or if you are obese (20 percent above normal weight). You should check your breasts during a regular monthly self-examination and have a yearly mammogram, but don't obsess. Statistics indicate that six times as many women die from heart disease than from breast cancer. And cancer caught early is treatable and curable. It has been well established that a lumpectomy in which the surgeon removes only the tumor and surrounding tissue plus radiation therapy is as effective as a mastectomy for women with an early stage of breast cancer.

CERVICAL CANCER

Women who have had multiple sex partners and/or use the Pill and smokers are at risk here. Don't skip a yearly Pap smear.

OVARIAN CANCER

If two or more close relatives had ovarian cancer, your risk is somewhat increased. Also at risk are those who have taken fertility drugs but never conceived. Even if your family medical history doubles your risk, the chances of developing this cancer are still only 2.8 percent. Since it's difficult to diagnose in its early stages, a yearly visit to your gynecologist is mandatory. And stay alert for and aware of any subtle changes or symptoms in your pelvic area.

COLON CANCER

Sometimes family background may be a contributor. A history of polyps bears watching. After forty we should have a rectal exam yearly; after fifty, a sigmoidoscopy every three to five years; and, if at risk, a colonoscopy every three to five years. Yes, it's a pain in the butt, but early discovery and treatment can save our lives. That's well worth the discomfort.

Skin Cancer

Those who have suffered from repeated sunburns, especially as a child, may be at risk, and so are those with light hair, light eyes, fair skin, freckles, or multiple moles. After fifty, years of exposure to the sun will be reflected in wrinkles and spots. Any inherited predisposition to precancerous lesions may show up. See a dermatologist every one to two years—or immediately if a mole or lesion changes color or shape.

A good relationship with a doctor whom we can trust is never more important than when we are diagnosed with cancer or any other serious illness. She or he will help you decide on treatment. We must feel comfortable discussing all our options with doctors who will support our choices.

An Inside Story

Is it gas or liver failure? Acidity or appendicitis? Do we need Tums for the tummy or a CAT scan? Stomach distress can be difficult to diagnosis, especially if it's a self-diagnosis.

Our inside organs are a mystery. Unlike our skin, the body's largest and very visible organ, most of us would have trouble locating our gallbladder. I have a vague notion that my liver and appendix are on the right and my kidneys are toward the back of that otherwise unchartered field that falls under the domain of an internist.

While I may not know the exact location of my inside organs, one really great benefit of having lived so long is that I've really gotten to know how my body reacts. And I understand how the general area that I refer to as my stomach will or won't cope with stress, overeating, too much fat, acid, or rich food, a stomach flu, an allergic reaction, or food poisoning.

Fatty foods can cause enough tummy trouble to convince me that I'm terminal. Coming from a long line of hypochondriacs, I do fret about and follow up on any egregious acid, bowel discomfort, excessive burping, or grumbling gas. If my stomach distress lasts longer than two weeks, I go to the doctor—though the symptoms seldom linger that long. A few years ago one seemingly fatal gas condition—what my grandmother Etta always referred to as a bilious attack and treated with home remedies: blueberry brandy or rhubarb and soda mixture—did disturb me for almost three weeks. While I was convinced this had to be "it," it wasn't.

Again, make certain you have a judicious, caring doctor who knows your insides better than you do, who listens to and respects your opinions, and who wouldn't hesitate to schedule a visit with a specialist. Consultation is good for the soul. God knows no one is thrilled to go through a GI series or can't wait to have a CAT scan or a barium enema, but sometimes those tests are necessary for an early diagnosis and effective treatment of what could be a serious condition. More likely what you'd feared was kidney pain that would no doubt lead to renal failure will turn out to be slight back strain.

A WOW should think of her doctor and herself as players on a winning team in the game of life. Choose your doctor with as much care as you'd choose a husband.

Our Doctors: How to Manage Their Care

HMO too often seems to stand for Hurried Medical Opinion. Any doctor who greets me juggling several charts and then keeps looking at his watch while taking my medical history is too harried to be my primary care physician. And I really resent sitting in an examination room wearing nothing but a paper hospital gown while a well-suited doctor is asking me questions whose answers obviously are boring him. Even if my health care provider is scheduled to see a certain number of patients per hour, doesn't his HMO provide him with desk space? The first step in becoming a team player with your doctor should be mutual respect. Therefore, it is not unreasonable to expect that a first consultation should require both the doctor and the patient to be fully clothed and seated in an office.

Call me chauvinistic, but my preferred primary care provider always has been a woman. Who wants to discuss hemorrhoids resulting from childbirth with some guy? And it doesn't matter how many letters he has after his name.

Six Steps to Selecting a WOW's Equally Wonderful Doctor

1. Prescreen the candidates. Finding the right doctor-patient partnership is like finding the right husband-wife partnership: It requires effort. If you're in the market for a new primary care physician, do your homework. Poll your friends and acquaintances, asking why they like their doctor. You'll be surprised how many people can't answer that question. The truth is they don't like their doctor but dislike change more. When you hear "He/she really listens to me!" put that doctor on your list of candidates. Some HMOs have an 800 number that new members can call, and, amazingly, a live person answers and gives a verbal biography about the PCPs available in your area.

My move to Washington, D.C., necessitated a switch in health insurance. After I'd narrowed my list of possible primary care providers to three, I called my new insurer's hot line and selected my doctor based on the information I heard. I'm delighted with her. However, if your first visit to your carefully chosen doctor turns out to be a disaster worse than your first blind date, you have the option in most plans to change your primary care physician. Exercise it!

2. Set forth your expectations during the first visit. Do your part to establish a comfortable relationship based on mutual respect. Don't be afraid to speak up about what you expect and need from a doctor-patient partnership. Women over fifty must make sure that their annual visits include a complete physical with an EKG as part of an ongoing health maintenance program. The primary care doctor should also provide referrals for cancer screenings (breast, gynecological, colon, and skin) and an eye exam. A woman who wants to be involved in the management of any health problems that may arise needs to discuss this during her first visit.

3. Come prepared and report symptoms in depth. You know the routine: On a first visit you're asked to give a complete medical history. If you're concerned about recalling the dates of any previous disease, illness, or operation; the related medical histories of your siblings, parents, and grandparents; or when you ceased menstruating, write it all down. Err on the side of including too much information rather than too little. And don't forget to bring your notes with you!

Even if your appointment is for a routine annual checkup, during that first office visit—before your examination—discuss all your symptoms and concerns in depth. For example, prolonged stiffness in one hand might be arthritis, but which type? Osteoarthritis, degenerative joint disease, affects almost 16 million mostly older Americans. And rheumatoid arthritis affects another 2 million, more than two-thirds of them women.

We owe it to ourselves and to our doctors to explain our current concerns, and our doctors owe us enough time to provide us with a complete explanation of the diagnosis, treatment, and prognosis.

4. Be totally truthful. There is no good reason to keep from your doctor any information that is even remotely related to your long-term good health, either during the first consultation or if your situation changes over time. As with a priest during confession, there is nothing you can say that would shock a doctor. He/she has heard it all before—and then some. So fess up regarding your current or past lifestyle, including smoking, drinking, drug use, or unsafe sex. Battered women and victims of incest should discuss those issues with the doctor so he/she can provide immediate advice and counsel.

5. Ask questions and offer opinions. Become an informed consumer. Ask for an explanation of any unfamiliar medical terms. Read up on any medical condition you may have and stay abreast of the latest treatments and new drugs. Use your acquired knowledge to offer informed opinions. Respect your doctor's judgment just as he/she should respect yours. Only then can you make an informed decision together.

6. Accept responsibility for your own past and future health choices. In the final analysis each of us is responsible for her own health. If a change in lifestyle is not just suggested but mandated, carefully consider the options. A wise WOW would welcome the second chance!

Life Beyond Menopause

I could have saved myself hours and hours of
worrying with one trip to the doctor!
   —A woman going through menopause

The six stages of a woman's life include childhood, puberty, reproductive maturity, menopause, postmenopause, and old age. The first three are history, menopause is a segue, and the last two are our future roles. Grim? Maybe—if that's what a woman's attitude toward aging is. But menopause is just an indicator that a woman has arrived at another plateau in her life cycle. It's not a disease or a delicate condition; rather, it's a natural passage that all women go through. And the last two stages of our lives can provide the best parts we've ever played. Menopause is "a transition rather than a trauma," as Judith Reichman, a gynecologist, said on the *Today Show.*

The average age for our last period is fifty-one. Menopause—the change from the reproductive stage to the postmenopause stage—can happen swiftly or can take as long as ten years!

Perimenopause, whose symptoms can include heavier, lighter, or skipped periods and sometimes hot flashes and vaginal dryness, can start years before periods stop. When a woman has not had a period for twelve consecutive months, she is considered to have gone through menopause.

I remember not having my period for three months when I was forty-six, in the middle of my longest (eleven years) and most serious relationship—actually, the love affair of my life. With a confirmed bachelor! I'd been worried that I might wind up as the oldest single mother in the world. A visit to the doctor assured me I wasn't pregnant, and my period arrived that very night, brought on either by the internal exam or extreme relief. Although my period continued to play hide-and-seek for the next five years, it totally vanished right on schedule when I was fifty-one.

So I've been officially postmenopausal for years. The trick is to survive the trip, which can have plenty of rough patches—not to mention hot spots. However, since Eve, centuries of women have moved beyond menopause unscathed, assuring us that this mental, emotional, physical, and in some ways spiritual journey can be successfully navigated. And the destination can be freedom!

"What? Menopause? I guess I was just too busy to notice!" said a post-menopausal *Foxy Forever* interviewee. Unlike that stoic WOW, I noticed plenty. At the onset of menopause I was working in Manhattan as the director of admissions at a small postsecondary school located in the Chrysler Building.

My daily "uniform" consisted of a smart, well-tailored little wool suit, often an Ellen Tracy, and a silk blouse. I'm here to tell you that hot flashes almost destroyed my winter wardrobe. I'd be on the phone or counseling a student when suddenly I'd sweat so profusely that my blouse would cling to my back and drops of perspiration would drip from my forehead. Since my job description included addressing assemblies of high school juniors and seniors, discussing a woman's role in the business world, I really sweated that sweat. I switched to cotton blouses and never went anywhere without shields and tons of tissues.

Yet somehow my psyche and my attitude weathered the heat waves a hell of a lot better than my body temperature.

While a small percentage of the women I questioned said that they'd experienced moderate to big-time depression, most said they had not. And while most certainly "noticed" and were irked by the flashes and other symptoms, they were indeed too busy living their lives to spend a lot of time dwelling on their changing bodies.

Running Hot and Cold and Other Menopausal Symptoms

Hot flashes are the second most common symptom of menopause after the changes in our periods. The flush of heat is often followed by chills; however, sometimes those chills precede the flashes. If the change in your period is manifested by heavy bleeding, that can be tough to manage, but it's usually a "normal" menopausal occurrence. Tell your doctor so he/she can make sure the bleeding doesn't stem from some other problem. With the decrease in estrogen, women often experience other symptoms: night sweats and vaginal changes, such as thinning, shrinking, and the previously mentioned dryness, which often can result in diminished sexual activity and pleasure. There is also an increased risk of getting vaginal or bladder infections. Not exactly a bed of roses, right? And we haven't even touched on the long-term health effects: Lower amounts of estrogen can mean a greater risk of heart disease and osteoporosis.

SUGGESTED TREATMENTS

Just as estrogen, or the lack of it, is the culprit, an infusion of that hormone combined with progesterone has become the panacea for most menopausal miseries. Estrogen is well established as the most effective way to prevent osteoporosis and heart disease.

In another appearance on the *Today Show*, Dr. Judith Reichman reported the results of new research which indicated that taking estrogen also may improve memory. Women who took the hormone experienced increased activity in the oxygen flow to and from the part of the brain used for storage of short memory, and it performs like a younger brain. The patients praised the improvement in their memories. One said, "I'm not searching for words."

Estrogen isn't recommended for everyone entering menopause. If a woman is worried about taking hormones because of her own medical problems or a family history of breast cancer, the gynecologist and the patient must evaluate the benefits and the risks.

Some women on estrogen complained to me about still getting artificially induced periods. More swear it's the fountain of youth. My friend Doris, the nurse, at first antiestrogen, started on it because of suffering extreme discomfort from hot flashes and sweats, but within a year she decided against the therapy.

More than a decade ago, with less known of the long-term results of estrogen therapy, I decided against taking any hormones. Now, at some risk for osteoporosis, I am on the estrogen Prempro and doing great, and my vaginal dryness is history.

Estrogen cream or an estrogen ring inserted in the vagina, both safe for high-risk women, are also options. Furthermore, research indicates that frequent sexual intercourse may improve lubrication and keep vaginal muscles toned. Since eventually we are all going to take DHEA and live to 105 while remaining "young at heart," that's great news!

For the Soul

Faith, hope, and love. As

Wonderful Older Women we

keep our spirits high, accept who

we are now, and celebrate each

day of our lives!

People Who Need People

Frankly, my dears, give a damn! That's what friends are for—giving and receiving emotional support. Who would you call at two o'clock in the morning when you're feeling like the wreck of the Hesperus and need someone to assure you that you're not? I call a friend from Category A, an exclusive group of three.

There are plateaus of friendship. You'd never call a friend from Category C—old school chums, your neighbors, your kids' friends' moms, or members of your bridge or Scrabble club—in the middle of the night to cry the blues. You'd select someone from the A list.

In the friendship game it's important to match the right people to the right category and not constantly crisscross categories. We can lose a pal that way—a perfectly good player who is forced to retreat from the game because of our too great expectations.

Though a C could never, sometimes a B friend moves up to an A. However, an A seldom slips down to a B. Like old soldiers, they either die or just fade away.

How It Works

The language of friendship is not words, but meanings. It is an intelligence above language.
—Thoreau

While all three categories are important to your friendship lifeline as well as your heart line, A is vital. Every WOW deserves at least two Category A people in her corner at all times, ready to stand by her side under any circumstances. Playing and winning, using the categories correctly, takes some practice.

The trick is to identify an A early on, separating her or him—a man might be a contender, but not often—from the rest of the competition.

THE RULES FOR MAINTAINING FOXY FOREVER FRIENDSHIPS

Rule One.   This is an equal opportunity game. On this board both you and your Category A friend must remain lifetime winners. Choose carefully. Don't let pride block your strategy. Don't make your move based on money, power, or charm, but if the right person possesses those three attributes, it's certainly a plus. An A list decision affects us forever. Only the wise, the witty, and the warm should make your A list. There's nothing like a sense of humor during a crisis; however, there's no room for chronic complainers, basic bores, torrid tempers, or the determinedly depressed. An A is the person you call in the middle of that miserable night, right? A friend who will listen and, except in extraordinary circumstances, give advice only when asked—or when you really need to hear it! Reciprocity is implicit in this deal. We're there, on call, for our Category A friends as well. That's one of the reasons two or three A's are the most we can handle.

Although a few who know me well have called me a QUIP (Queens Irish Princess), in general, princesses are not the best choices for Category A, though they can be a great challenge and lots of fun when used to fill in the blanks in Category B.

Rule Two.   Offer unconditional love and supply emotional support even if you disapprove of how your friend is playing her cards.

How can your bright, beautiful best friend still be dating that married man? The one who has been on the verge of a divorce for the last twenty-two years? You think he's a slime bucket, and though you hate to admit it, she's a damn fool. How well you handle those feelings of outrage can determine if you remain in each other's Category A.

Rule Three. Total acceptance. So she's gone and dyed her hair orange, is wearing a hat decorated with cherries, and her skirt is made of
spandex. She's an A. She's your friend. You picked her. Now either accept
her as she is or strike her from the A lineup. But be aware of one caveat:
Once a player has been removed from that category, she is probably out
of the game forever. We should never drop an A for a shallow reason; it's
difficult enough to drop one for serious cause. Under almost all circumstances, a friend who has earned an A deserves to keep it. And expect
no less from her.

Category A friends who break the rules can make us feel foolish or
furious. When an A doesn't live up to our expectations, it can be more
devastating then being betrayed by a husband or lover. That is why the
next rule is so important.

Rule Four. Be honest. Your Category A friendships deserve the
complete truth. This may be rather like tap dancing through a minefield,
but the more honest we are with each other, the more courageous we
become. Don't confuse honesty with criticism, cynicism, judgment, or
opinion. Remember that unsolicited criticism hurts. Sarcasm stings. And
don't believe that your truth is infallible—or even, necessarily, your
friend's truth.

Rule Five. Always treat your Category C people as you do your
Category B friends. You'll share many fun social occasions with them.
You'll reminisce with them at high school and college reunions. Your son
might even marry one of their daughters.

Rule Six. Cherish your Category B players. Respect them as much
as you do Category A friends. You never know when a B may accumulate
enough points to move up. A Category B friend often is someone whom
you've known for a long time, someone you trust, and someone whose
input you value. However, the spark that ignites intimacy isn't there. That
status can change—sometimes overnight. Sharing an unexpected joy,
common cause, or difficult time can turn a caring but possibly replaceable
B into an indispensable, loving A. Or maybe late one night while two
players from Category B are swapping old war stories, the chemistry simply explodes into an A friendship.

Forget About Foes

After fifty there is no time to harbor grudges, hang on to resentments, or have an emotional hit list. A wise WOW heeds Eleanor Roosevelt's advice: "No one can make you feel inferior without your consent."

Remember Friends

A true friend is one soul in two bodies.
                                                    —Aristotle

Sometimes a tragedy moves friends from a B to an A. In the mid-eighties I had two longtime A friends, Doris Holland and Mary Fahy Celeste. Both had been on my Category A short list for decades.

I was introduced to Mary, a beautiful blonde and funny as hell, at Rockaway Beach when we were teenagers. We shared showers, weddings, births, summer cottages, the funerals of our parents, Christmas holidays, our divorces, the children's college graduations, her remarriage, her second divorce, and, finally, the grim medical prognosis that without a liver transplant her illness would be terminal.

Doris and I met in the early sixties while spending a Labor Day holiday weekend at Lake George. Our crowd of young married couples had a tradition of closing out the summer waterskiing and partying in upstate New York while our parents baby-sat our kids. Doris, a chic French Canadian, had just ended an international romance and came along with one of the couples "to get over it." That same weekend she met her future husband, another member of our group who had just been divorced. And despite some strong reservations on my part, they were married nine months later. Doris and I had fallen in instant like at Lake George, and at the time of her wedding we were Category B friends. By the mid-seventies, when both of our marriages had ended, we had a very close long-standing Category A friendship.

With Mary's return to New York City after her second divorce, the three of us, together with our now almost grown-up children, spent most

Easter Sundays and all Christmas Eves together. Mary and Doris had resumed their Category B friendship. (Sometimes we won't see a B friend for years but remain close via letters, phone calls, and, today emails, a great information age gift to long-distance friendship.) Husbands and lovers came and went—no pun intended—but we three friends knew we could always count on one another.

Though we were working women, taking full responsibility for our own lives, we all suffered from the Cinderella Complex, the curse of most women who came of age in the late fifties and early sixties. We just kept looking for that damn white horse with Prince Charming in the saddle to trot up Madison Avenue, and we just kept getting splattered with dirty water from taxis that never stopped. Nevertheless, we had a hell of a lot of fun searching—at least most of the time.

Then in the mid-eighties the three of us were on a mini vacation at Xanadu. The geodesic dome on Lake Champlain was the home of our friend Janine, the same one who had taken care of me after my lift, and her husband, Ken. In the bright February morning's sunlight, as we ski-walked on the frozen lake, Doris, the never-really-off-duty nurse, noticed that Mary's eyes were yellow. So was her skin.

Two weeks later I waited in Mary's room at New York Hospital while she, insisting on going it alone, met with the doctors for the results of her weeklong intensive and invasive tests. The diagnosis was a relatively rare but very serious liver disease that had advanced far enough to clog Mary's bile ducts. The doctors discussed the possibility of a transplant. What they didn't tell her that morning was that without a transplant she'd die.

In 1984 liver transplants were fairly new procedures, smacking somewhat of science fiction. At first Mary wouldn't consider that option. She still felt pretty good, and with the right color makeup and dark glasses covering her eyes, she looked great. No one could tell that she was jaundiced.

Her three kids—actually young adults—had no idea how sick their mother was. She had forbidden us to tell them, and I don't think she believed it herself.

That April, Mary said, "Let's have a big Easter dinner at my apartment; everyone can bring something." And we did.

"We have to get through Ronald's graduation from West Point first," she said in May. "We'll have a luncheon, and that night we'll celebrate with a big party in Manhattan." And we did.

"Wait until the summer is over, and then I promise to talk about the transplant option. Meantime, let's spend a long weekend on Shelter Island." And we did.

But by her birthday in October, feeling physically tired and even more tired of listening to Doris and me nagging her, Mary agreed to discuss a transplant with her doctor. Pittsburgh's waiting list was too long, so he suggested the Mayo Clinic where a Dutch doctor was having some wonderful results. Mary wanted to wait until after Christmas. And we did.

Thinking it might help her move faster, I accompanied Mary to a PBC (Primary Biliary Cirrhosis) support group. In New York City, no matter how obscure the illness, you can find a support group. The ravages of the disease were visible on the faces of three of the five women in attendance. Mary, however, looked better than I did. I'm sure that they assumed I, a total wreck, was the patient. One woman had a beeper, waiting for her transplant call. Another had resigned herself to death. Her insurance didn't cover a transplant, and she had no money. A third in the early stages of PBC had her husband with her. Suspecting what the diagnosis might turn out to be, he had upped her insurance to the max and was paying sky-high premiums.

We left the meeting feeling totally confused and frightened. Fortunately, Mary worked as a legal secretary for a large law firm in Rockefeller Center and had excellent health insurance.

But she remained adamant that if this was to be her last Christmas, she damn well wanted to celebrate it with her kids in New York. She made arrangements to go to Minnesota for a liver transplant evaluation in January.

Christmas Eve was less than merry. Mary arrived looking thin; her arms and legs, always slender, were now skinny; and her stomach, full of fluid, was horribly bloated. She looked like those pictures of third world babies, dying from starvation. And she could no longer deny to her children that she was very ill.

Doris insisted that she stay with her until she felt better. For a while Mary divided her time between the Hollands' and home. She tried to go back to work but couldn't. In early January, Doris, my friend John, and I drove Mary to the airport for her flight to the Mayo Clinic.

She stayed there ten days, and I guess the doctors pulled no punches. Mary called crying, "If I don't have a transplant within six months, I'll be dead." However, they couldn't operate even if they had a liver. The varicose veins on her legs needed work; the doctors were concerned about possible infection. In those early days of liver transplants, the surgeons sweated the statistics; they wanted to ensure the success of their operations. Mary returned to Manhattan for treatment on her veins.

In a decision not up for negotiation, Doris moved Mary, bag and baggage, into her house and set her up in her daughter's room. Doris and her two children, Jennifer and JP, took care of her. In the beginning, Mary would have a cocktail ready and the table set when Doris returned from work, but then a bleeding episode put her in the local hospital. She almost died; she was out of it and lost an entire day, hovering between life and death. She would have died if JP hadn't come home from school and found her on the bathroom floor. Doris brought her home from the hospital to nurse her. No patient ever had more TLC. We all agreed that as soon as Mary regained a modicum of strength, we'd try again for a transplant.

Two weeks later Mary and I left for the Mayo Clinic. I stayed for several days—thanks to God and a compassionate boss—and Mary remained and prepared for the transplant—if they located a liver.

Mary was so sick on the plane that the stewardess moved us up front, swathed her in blankets, and arranged for a wheelchair to be available at the arrival gate so we could make the connecting flight. She suggested having an ambulance waiting in Minneapolis, but I insisted that we go on to Rochester. We both thought that Mary might not last the flight.

Once ensconced in the Mayo Clinic, Mary rallied. She apologized for and joked about scaring me to death. But the doctors, while cheering

Mary on, told me her kidneys were failing. Other organs appeared damaged as well. A transplant was looking less likely. The internist heading the team told me that her chances were not good, that other candidates were in better overall health. And I knew time was running out.

On the day I left, Mary felt pretty good, and the doctors seemed more optimistic. However, she did gave me a list of instructions for her funeral and for the distribution of her Wedgwood "just in case." I departed feeling cautiously optimistic.

Janine flew out to be with Mary, arriving on the day they extracted all her teeth—for fear of infection—in preparation for surgery. They still had no liver. And Mary still had problems. But if they took the trouble to pull her teeth . . .

I called Mary and said, "They're waiting for the perfect liver. Maybe we can hire a hit man to knock off Marie Osmond," I joked. "She's never even had a drink!"

Doris flew out, taking Mary's daughter, Maggi, with her. Every night Doris called me with messages of hope. Finally, she had to go back to work.

The social worker insisted that Mary allow her to call her oldest son; Mary had tried to protect her kids to the very end. Ronald arrived just before his mother died. His sister met him at the hospital. Gregg, though ready to go, never made it.

The next day, Easter Sunday, Doris and I had dinner at my sister's. Doris had spoken to Mary that morning. She had been put on morphine. Though I remained in denial, we all knew this would be it, that once a patient went on drugs, there could be no transplant. Mary died the next morning.

When the social worker called to express her sorrow—she had really liked Mary and had been rooting for her—she told me Mary not only knew she was dying but had accepted it. "One of the last things she said to me was 'It's okay. I'm going to have a cup of tea with my mother in heaven.' Then she smiled."

Doris and I tucked two Lipton tea bags into Mary's casket.

Over the last few years Mary's two grandchildren, her son Ronald's darling little boys, as well as their mom and dad and Aunt Maggi and

Uncle Gregg, in keeping with our extended family tradition, have spent Christmas Eve at Doris's home. All of our grown children have stayed in touch; my son, Billy, sees a good deal of Ronald, Lucina, and the boys. And when we all get together, we often swap Mary stories. I like to think that somewhere up there she's still smiling.

When Irish Eyes
Are Smiling

Growing up as an Irish Catholic was both weird and wonderful, not unlike the mysteries of the Rosary: joyful, sorrowful, and glorious. You finished five decades, and you switched emotions on cue. We just did it, switched emotions, I mean, but we have never talked about them. Feelings, like lasagne, were something Italian families had.

What the Irish had were secrets. "Don't tell the neighbors. And for God's sake don't tell your father" were the eleventh and twelfth commandments in my house—especially if I had broken one of the original ten.

But then I was well schooled in secrets and sacrifice, incense and innocence, penance and prayers, sinners and saints, virgins and martyrs and sainted virgin martyrs, mite boxes and Mystery. Mystery with a capital "M."

QUESTION: "Sister, how can there be three persons in one God?"

ANSWER: "That's the Divine Mystery of the Holy Trinity. God the Father, God the Son, and God the Holy Ghost." (The latter hadn't as yet undergone a name change to the Holy Spirit.)

QUESTION: "Sister, how can we be sure that all of us practicing Catholics are going to get into heaven when all those unbaptized babies are going to limbo for eternity?" (That seemed like a hell of a long time for my ten-year-old mind to comprehend.)

ANSWER: "Why, Noreen, you know that's a Mystery of Faith."
QUESTION: "Sister, but . . ."
ANSWER: "You have been chosen, baptized into the one true Roman
Catholic faith. Jesus died on the cross for you. You are a temple of the
Holy Ghost. Why are you questioning God's gift? Pray for the renewal of
your faith, my child. Recite the glorious mysteries of the Rosary."

> *May you be in heaven a half-hour before the devil*
> *knows you're gone.*
>   —An Irish toast

The home fires were burning, too. Since hell was not an option, as
a family we all went to Mass every Sunday and daily during Lent. We
observed fast days. Made novenas. Took the annual Legion of Decency
pledge, swearing not to attend suggestive or subversive movies. We also
attended missions, which were often led by hell, fire, and brimstone
preachers straight from the Elmer Gantry school-of-thought seminary.
Single women were segregated from married women, and we were all
segregated from the men. As ordained by Saint Margaret Mary, we received Holy Communion on the first Fridays of nine consecutive months
and sometimes, in honor of Our Lady of Fatima, on the first Saturdays,
praying for a plenary indulgence—kind of a free pass out of hell or a
shorter sentence in purgatory—for ourselves and for the souls of our
dearly departed.

Ours was an extended family—multiple generations, not additions
and substractions of sundry stepsiblings. When my mother married my
father, he came as a package deal, so I was blessed and cursed with three
role models, wise and witty women: my great-grandmother, Anastasia
Walsh Donnelly; Gran, my grandmother, Loretta Donnelly Feeley, known
as Etta; and my marvelous mother, Nora Guiney Feeley.

Through all my school years I never once came home to an empty
house. I came home to an attentive audience, Milky Ways sliced and
arranged on a doily or white bread with crust trimmed and topped with
a dollop of butter and a smidgen of sugar, accompanied by a "nice" cup
of tea—real tea steeped in a cozy-covered pot and served in a china cup.

At was liberally laced with milk and love. In school the solution often seemed to be faith, but in our home, no matter what the problem, putting on the kettle was the answer. It seemed easier to accept or understand the slings and arrows of outrageous classmates while savoring tea and sympathy, especially when brewed by a feisty Irish-American grandmother and poured by a supportive mother.

I also had a beautiful, bright, well-behaved older sister, Helen, a tough act to follow. Since I was bold, a constant chatterbox, and spoiled silly, I became the scourge of the good sisters, starting in the first grade. As a consequence, my mother spent a considerable amount of time "in conference" with my teachers and Sister Superior regarding my "high spirits" and my term-after-term "C" in conduct. Of course, we never told my father.

My father thought he was God, and since the women in his life treated him as if he were, that seemed to work. Youthful, compact, and handsome, with a boyish grin and silver hair, he played ragtime piano, was quick to anger and quicker to laugh, mixed old-fashioneds with all the solemnity of the consecration of the Mass, drove us to the beach every summer Saturday, took all of us away for an August and sometimes a winter holiday, worked as a fast-rising executive at an oil company, was always after me to clean my fingernails and stand up straight, and held court every night. When he caught me roller-skating in the street, I had to stand in a corner for an hour. And I couldn't skate for a week. But on most occasions when I was grounded, my grandmother, defying his orders, would take me out for an ice cream soda. I never knew what to say to him and never had an in-depth conversation with him, though he called every day when I went to the hospital with whooping cough. Sometimes I think I was afraid of him; other times I think I resented him because when he came home, he stole all the attention away from me.

He expected much, but he asked little. The only advice I can ever recall Bill Feeley giving me was posed in the form of a teasing question, usually on the way home from the beach: "Do you know why you have to keep your eyes open?" Then he'd answer it for me. "If you don't, you can't see anything."

Set thine house in order.

—II Kings 20:1

When they weren't busy not telling my father anything that might incur his displeasure, discomfort, or dismay, the Feeley women were busy cleaning. No commercial laundry has ever gotten my shirts as white as my mother did. Washing—using a scrub board until we bought a washing machine—was an all-day affair. Bleaching, bluing, starching, then hanging out to dry. We may not have aired our dirty laundry, but we certainly filled the line with our clean linen. This was followed by folding and ironing.

Etta's specialties included the entrance hall and the bathroom that five of us used every day. The tub always gleamed, the mirror and glass shone, and the tile had no grit. I think her secret (there's that word again) weapon was a combination of ammonia, lye, and brown soap. More than one friend told me that our vestibule smelled like a doctor's operating room.

All will come out in the wash.

—Cervantes

Simmering in that Irish stew, sprinkled with secrets, stirred by sad songs of young soldiers, and peppered with large slices of blarney, was a good dose of common sense. As I grow older, and with almost a lifetime spent rebelling against it, my grandmother's advice, "Don't air your dirty laundry," no longer seems arcane.

After decades of watching most of us—including me—let it all hang out so the immediate world could see, hear, and wallow in our soiled linen, I've decided that Etta may have been right. Indeed, I now believe her advice could have helped me through this last half-century if I hadn't chosen to ignore it.

We've been sidetracked over the years by other options: EST, psychodrama, Hair Pullers Anonymous, group therapy, General Confession, and Jerry Springer. My grandmother would be appalled. She was washed and starched at all times, literally and figuratively.

Maybe it's time for us to allow some old-fashioned restraint to reenter our collective consciousness and to give ourselves a swift kick in our overanalyzed butts.

Confession may be good for the soul. And as a girl who made those nine first Fridays so often that it's guaranteed Saint Margaret Mary and the entire host of angels will greet me at heaven's gate, I certainly blabbed like a regular Irish yenta long before confessing to the masses became hot segments on trashy television talk shows. A maverick among my close-mouthed family, who never bared either their bodies or their souls to each other, I could confide with the greatest of ease. However, I'm now convinced too much sharing of our private lives with anyone who'll listen can leave us emotionally bankrupt, not to mention turn us into bloody bores.

While they told my father and the neighbors nothing, my mother and grandmother were always asking me—particularly if I was loud, looked slovenly, or engaged in a fight with another little kid—"What will your father say?" or "What will the neighbors think?"

Like most childhoods, mine was full of mixed messages. But then sometimes I think my entire life has been a mixed message.

Can a Member of Our Own Family Ever Turn into a Category A Player?

If my niece had been born two days later, she would have been Patricia; instead, my sister checked out which saint celebrated her feast day on March 15 and called her daughter Susan.

Though I had not yet received my Confirmation, through some sort of special dispensation three weeks later, wearing my Easter outfit and totally thrilled, I became Susan's godmother.

Flash-forward fifty years. Why am I in Washington? Last March 15 I came to help Susan move. I fell in love with the wonderful old landmark building, and, tired of sand in my shoes, decided to leave Florida and move in there, too. Two months later, eighteen boxes and I arrived at Susan's lovely co-op and stayed for three months while I waited for an apartment. No one but a Category A player could put up with that move. Actually, I chose D.C. for three reasons: I wanted to live in a city, but Manhattan had become too pricey. I love Washington: It's so pretty and only a shuttle ride to New York. And most important in my game plan, my Category A niece/friend lives there, right in the same apartment house!

A final thought: You know you've succeeded as a mom when your son or daughter makes your A list of friends. Billy—yes, named for my father—has made mine. And, thank God, I believe it's reciprocal.

What Are You Doing the Rest of Your Life?

Will you *Whistle While You Work*, will you enroll for *School Days, School Days*, will you go *Around the World in Eighty Days*, or will you stay home and, as a grandparent, reprise your role as a mother for *The Second Time Around*?

About one-fourth of the Wonderful Older Women told me that they'll never retire—some because they love what they do, more because they'd go crazy not working, but even more because they need the money. I fit into all those categories.

World-Weary Women in the Workplace

"Put it in inside out and upside down," my thirty-one-year-old-going-on-thirteen boss instructed me.

"That's the story of my life," I replied.

He looked just like Opie if Opie had grown up to look the way I'd always imagined he would instead of turning into Ron Howard. We were staring at the printer attached to my ACT-programmed state-of-the-art computer. As far as ACT was concerned, I'd been listening to the overture while Opie had been taking curtain calls. An icon to him was a tiny tool on a monitor. An icon to me was a saint or at least a plastic replica of one. Generation X versus a world-weary woman.

Knowing when to retreat, I quit. I hadn't liked the job all that much, and I'd liked Opie even less. And my first book would be coming out that summer. Opie may have thought he'd won the battle against the older woman in the workplace. I believed I'd won the war, though I'd gone against all sound advice by giving up my day job to become a full-time writer. Since over two years went by before I had another contract and advance, it may have been a Pyrrhic victory. The major casualty turned out to be the loss of a steady income, an occupational hazard that many writers suffer from but seem to survive. Maybe we who write for a living are all a little crazy.

My checkered careers have included fashion, education, television, sales, management, and being the oldest model in New Jersey. Maybe I switched direction so frequently because I was searching for the right path, the one that would keep me happy and on track. However long and roundabout, my journey finally led me to where I should have been all along.

Being an author is not only the career that I've dreamed of having since I read my first Nancy Drew book, but it's the best one yet. I get to create my job description because I'm my own boss and make my own hours. My only discipline is a deadline, but that's more than enough motivation. I'm writing as fast as I can. And it's *murder!* The first book in my Ghostwriter mystery series, starring Jake O'Hara, arrived in the bookstores in June 1999. The second, *Death Comes for the Critic*, in February 2000. Jake and I both love murder and mayhem, and writing at home I can continue to plot as long as my imagination remains alive and deadly.

A SECOND CHANCE FOR A GREAT CAREER

Wonderful Older Women are accepting new challenges in new fields, many saying that the later-in-life career changes are like transfusions of energy empowering them to remain foxy forever.

Marti Smye's book, *Is it Too Late to Run Away and Join the Circus? Finding the Life You Really Want*, asks and answers the question. As Smye points out, Wonderful Older Women have some very good reasons to consider a career change:

> They hate the job.
> They are forced out.
> They need to continue working because the Social Security benefit age keeps going higher and higher.

If you're bored after twenty years in the same career, Smye advises, "Don't be ashamed to admit it. Test-drive a second career." She cites the example of a teacher who went to work during a summer vacation at a bed-and-breakfast thinking she'd like to open one, only to discover that she didn't like making beds. If you can't take a summer off, make every effort to try out your possible new career on weekends. Ask yourself what you love to do on your own time, what you're really passionate about. Then figure out how you can get paid to do it.

I agree. Do you want out? Deeply? Madly? Truly? Hey, this is your life, the only one you have. Admit it to yourself. Then tell your family, your Category A friends, and, when you've done your homework and faced your future, your boss.

REDEFINING OUR OFFICES

Chances are, whether you grab a subway and head downtown to work in a skyscraper or create in a small corner of your house, your office will no longer be a room with four walls, elegant wood furnishings, an impressive desk, and a window with a great view. Tradition has been replaced by technology. In the workplace this has resulted in employers utilizing smaller spaces and smaller staffs but expecting higher productivity. With over 60 million Americans working at home, the space that we now refer to as an office can range from a computer workstation tucked into a nook in the den to a laptop on a dining room table or a cell phone in a car.

In this brave, new, portable world, what you do has become more important than who you are. And as Martha Stewart would say, that's a good thing. Flexibility in hours and job site as well as a new definition of what is a typical employee are all advantages for a career-changing WOW.

ARE THE RULES DIFFERENT FOR WOMEN OVER FIFTY?

In our later-in-life second or third careers, most of us probably wouldn't choose to walk into a boardroom filled with thirty-something guys who might consider us relics and treat us like their mothers. However, if we do opt for a corporate position, we must be prepared to meet the challenges of a working WOW in the twenty-first century with confidence, enthusiasm, and energy.

Rosalie Bernstein, with twenty years experience in placement, says, "Many companies prefer to hire mature employees because their track records have shown better attendance, better attitudes, and better on-the-job performance. I have no problem placing people over fifty. Their skills and experience are their strengths, even in a highly competitive marketplace."

Our society puts far too much emphasis on youth and beauty rather than on brains and experience, and this prejudice often spills over into corporate America. Several successful women told me that blatant age discrimination had sent them scurrying to a plastic surgeon. There are many excellent reasons to have cosmetic surgery; job stress isn't one of them.

As Wonderful Older Women we should be the ones who discriminate, and if we decide to return to the corporate world, we should choose a company that values competent, experienced, well-groomed employees.

WHEN WORK IS A LIFELONG PASSION

There are Wonderful Older Women who have always loved their work and have no intention of either changing careers or ever retiring. Many of America's most productive women are now over sixty-five, performing in diverse positions—from caterers to CEOs, from realtors to reverends, from musicians to microbiologists.

Consider seventy-plus Barbara Walters. When does this ubiquitous WOW sleep? Dr. Joyce Brothers has been dishing out advice on television and in print for almost fifty years. She's currently in great demand as a "talking head." Debbie Reynolds has been acting, dancing, and singing since the late forties, both in the rain and on the soundstage, and remains a multifaceted star in movies, television, and the theater. The feminine feminist Gloria Steinem, in her late sixties, is going strong, preaching to a new generation while reminding all of us that our paychecks should have more to do with skill than sex. Or our age. Sexy and over seventy, cabaret star Eartha Kitt keeps purring those torch songs. And at eighty journalist Helen Thomas, the dean of the White House press corps, continues to ask the toughest and most intelligent questions. I chatted with Helen a few years ago at a Chamber of Commerce breakfast in Fort Lauderdale, and I can assure you that this WOW will stay a front-runner on the foxy forever career track.

But the WOW "Hi Ho, Hi Ho, It's Off to Work We Go Award" goes to Audrey Stubbart, just another working gal who, as an over-one-hundred-year-old great-great-grandmother, is still on the job! Audrey never took a day off during her fifty-plus years as a proofreader for the *Examiner*, a daily newpaper in Independence, Missouri. Stubbart said that if she called in, she wouldn't be sick, she'd be dead. A lady who loved her work!

Many of us do. And like these Wonderful Older Women, we have from day one. If we can, we'll work forever. I must admit, though, that I sometimes suffer from a relapse of the Cinderella syndrome and wish I had *Someone to Watch Over Me*. Someone really rich!

Fit for Service: From Miss Subway to Capitol Hill to Fitness Trainer

With clippings from *Roll Call* and an American Senior Fitness Association press release reporting on her new career as a personal trainer, Eleanor Nash-Brown is a well-publicized WOW! The fifty-seven-year-old's fledgling but already extremely successful enterprise, Fit and Healthy Forever, serves as an example for other Wonderful Older Women who are considering a career change and/or are dreaming of opening their own business. Eleanor also serves as a role model for having a strong, toned body at any age.

"An older woman feels more comfortable developing a fitness program and working out with a trainer who is her peer" was Eleanor Nash-Brown's astute observation, and she began a fitness training program that led her to a career in overfifty fitness. "Some of my clients are over seventy, and as I watch them grow stronger and gain confidence, my own goals are reinforced. I love my work."

So what did it take to get started? Eleanor's answer: motivation and determination. Nash-Brown seems to have no shortage of either.

Growing up in the Bronx, Eleanor Nash-Brown had a brief modeling career and in the 1960s was a Miss Subways. I swear I remember seeing her pretty face—still lovely today—as I rode to work all those decades ago. She was also a contestant in the Miss New York Pageant. The latter brought her to Grossinger's in the Catskills. Eleanor liked Ulster County. "Why not? It was better than the Bronx!" She stayed upstate, married, and lived in Ellenville. When her two children were in nursery school, she started a petition to fight the local utility company's soaring rates. She wound up with over five thousand signatures, and, albeit unintentionally, her political career was born.

Eleanor recalls: "This was a time when women never discussed a 'career' or career goals. Mine just happened." Running for county legislator as a Democrat in an overwhelmingly Republican district, Nash-Brown won and served for two years. Climbing the political ladder, she then worked for the U.S. Congress for twenty years, beginning in 1978.

Like most of us, Eleanor had exercised in spurts over the years. About six years ago, she says, "stress drove me to work out! I got serious, joined the Washington Sports Club, a short walk from Capitol Hill, and began getting up at five-thirty, four mornings a week, to work out with a personal trainer and on the machines before I went to my office." Two things happened. "In a very short time I felt great, and I became convinced I'd like to help other women feel great." While preparing to retire as chief of staff for Congressman Maurice Hinchey, Eleanor spent two years juggling a most demanding job on the Hill and going to school to obtain her certification as a personal trainer.

Five months into her new career Eleanor has so many fifty-plus clients that she can make her own hours. Holding four certifications, she plans to continue her own fitness education and complete a certification in osteoporosis exercise and another with the College of Sports Medicine. Nash-Brown is considering a move to Fort Lauderdale to be near her mom and her son who is about to be married. (She also has a daughter in Atlanta.) Florida should prove a fertile field for a senior fitness expert.

Chronologically the oldest personal trainer at both health clubs where she works part-time, Eleanor Nash-Brown is a counselor, a role model, and an intrepid cheerleader for her clients. She spent part of our interview teaching me upper-arm exercises and offered to stop by my gym and show me more! Eleanor's energy, determination, and dedication make her an inspiration for any WOW who wants and deserves that second chance to turn her great passion into a great career.

As the boomers age, Wonderful Older Women in the workplace will play starring roles in America's future economy.

School Days,
School Days

If you're thinking about going back to school, don't fret about being the oldest student in the class. From adult ed to Ph.D. programs, Wonderful Older Women are enrolling and studying side by side with younger class-mates.

Grandma is a WordPerfect freshman. Count on her graduating with honors and getting her master's in Microsoft Excel. Her new skills will open "Windows" to new careers. Adults over fifty are among the fastest growing group of personal computer purchasers. If you're one of the few remaining people left in America who are not computer literate, you're in good company. You're with me. Even though when it comes to technology I'm the world champion procrastinator—usually I'm the type who jumps into the pool without taking a swimming lesson—I'm enrolling in a class this summer.

One finger on a word processor has proved to be less than an efficient way to produce a manuscript. More important, I want to get online and flood my friends with email. Since I'm an author who works alone and I haven't as yet found a Washington writing group, I'd like to be part of a writers' chat group. I've been told that a computer can be a companion. Taking that electronic step further, one work-at-home WOW met her second husband in a chat room.

Most of the Wonderful Older Women I interviewed have taken job-related computer classes and say that when they no longer want to work full-time, they can temp. And if that seems too ho-hum or if you don't want or need to work at all, you can go back to school. Take that class in Greek mythology, preferably in Athens or aboard a ship to Rhodes. Or mainstream in a college right in your hometown. Get that degree in English lit or study painting.

A Well-Rounded Working WOW

Barbara Crowley-Georgio of Farmington Hills, Michigan, was divorced after twenty-five years of marriage and stay-at-home momhood, with three teenagers in high school and one in college. Crowley-Georgio went back to college and received her B.S. in human services while working full-time and continuing to raise her children. When she was human resource coordinator at Botsford General Hospital, a grandmother, and taking care of her elderly aunt, Barbara returned to school to pursue a master's degree. Despite a three-year bout with a muscle inflammation disease, Barbara exudes energy, looks great, plays golf like a pro, travels extensively, and has the most active social life of all the Wonderful Older Women I interviewed.

School Trips

For Wonderful Older Women who are no longer working, it's good to know that Elder Hostel is getting younger. Several downsized-early and long-retired Wonderful Older Women raved about taking Elder Hostel classes, studying unusual subjects, and making new friends among their classmates in such great locations as the Grand Canyon, San Francisco, and Paris. Attending an Elder Hostel program is like auditing a college course with your peers. What a way to learn!

Living with Longevity

If it sounds as if I'm stressing that we should keep our bodies, souls, and minds active, it's because I am. In *The Longevity Factor*, Lydia Bronte, Ph.D., director of the Aging Society Project, a special study sponsored by the Carnegie Corporation of New York, discusses a second middle age from fifty to seventy-five, and old age starting later as a gift of time, allowing us to create a long career. The track of old age and retirement in our sixties has been derailed. Most of us have a lot of time ahead of us, not something to fear but a bonus.

Late bloomers will have a much longer time to blossom and grow in their new career of choice. Would anyone really want to be retired for over a quarter-century? Just how many golf and tennis games can we look forward to winning? So when you're ready to retire, if you feel you've worked long enough, I suggest that to stay foxy forever you should plan on some constructive time each day. If not a paid position, volunteer at a hospital or school and/or have a hobby that you love and that will keep you intellectually challenged.

Tenacity Plus Talent Multiplied by Purpose Equals Success

Artist Lois Jones, after seventy-five years of trying to gain recognition, now has her work hanging in such galleries as the Smithsonian's National Museum of American Art, the Metropolitan Museum of Art in New York, and the Museum of Fine Art in Boston. It really is never too late. Jones said, "At ninety I arrived." And the chief curator of the Corcoran Gallery of Art in Washington concurred. Quoted in the *AARP Bulletin,* Jack Cowart said, "Lois's name has entered the canon of noteworthy art of our time."

Hobby for Hire

While having a hobby that you love is a joy in itself, having a hobby that turns a profit provides a wondrous way to earn extra money. Selling paintings and pottery, teaching bridge or exercise classes, opening a gourmet bake shop—all across America, Wonderful Older Women are spinning their hobbies off into a successful second career, sometimes more successful than their first career.

"It's the love factor," Diane Dowling Dufour says. Already working part-time as a fashion and beauty consultant, Diane has started another late-in-life career. "I evolved into a wedding planner and interior decorating coordinator after decades of doing both jobs as kind of hobby at no charge for friends. Eventually their referrals to their friends paid for my services. But while the money is great, what I really love is the challenge of changing a barren room into a beautiful setting!"

Waking up and looking forward to working at what they love is the way many Wonderful Older Women have chosen to go. And when a hobby becomes a career, age is no barrier.

My Story

If I had a gun to my head and had to choose between reading or eating ice cream for the rest of my life, there would be no flinching. I'd opt for murder mysteries over hot fudge sundaes, though ideally I'd prefer to enjoy both concurrently.

In 1994 while living and working at a "real job" in Florida, I took a writing class. And another. Then I discovered Joyce Sweeney, who taught me point of view, plot turns, character development, and how to craft an opening scene and then chapter by chapter build to an unexpected climax. I had two ideas: a nonfiction book based on my stints as a contestant on seven different television game shows, and a murder mystery set at the Algonquin Hotel in New York City and starring the members of the Roundtable. The latter proved to be far too ambitious an undertaking for a neophyte. But after that five-week session with Joyce, she invited me and three other students to join her advanced class: a weekly writing/ critique workshop filled with talented, inspiring men and women of all ages and from diverse backgrounds and professions. I attended those workshops for two years and referred to those Thursday nights as "going to school."

I also began to attend local weekend writing conferences, especially those featuring New York agents as guest panelists. That's how I met Peter Rubie, my longtime agent. Following him down the hall, I pitched him the contestant idea. He said, "Send a proposal and sample chapter." Peter sold the book within a month, and my writing career took off.

Publishing is a capricious business filled with creative starts and stumbling blocks. My second proposal didn't sell so quickly. With no job and no advance, I agreed to work as a ghostwriter, hating every page and asking myself, "What fresh hell will each new client bring?" The book, a memoir, was based on the author's premise that the entire world was against her. An ex-husband was cast as the main villain, but her parents, siblings, children, country club members, and condo neighbors were all coconspirators. And though I really needed the money, by the third chapter I could have killed her myself.

What I hadn't realized at the time is that during that deadly assignment a seed was planted. Being a ghost led me to murder—writing about it, not committing it. And there's no mystery about it: My school days, all those writing classes and seminars, led to my current career as a mystery series author.

My fashion/modeling background, combined with my burning desire to put a fresh face on aging, led to *Foxy Forever*.

More and more Wonderful Older Women are discovering that their best careers are yet to come.

Around the World in Eighty Days

One of the best things about becoming a WOW—and I grant you that some days the list can appear mighty meager—is the discounts dished out by the travel industry. Your travel agent should be up to the minute on all such "senior" bargains, but too often finding the right travel agent can be as tough as finding the right psychiatrist or plastic surgeon. And as with any purchase, when selecting a vacation package, the decision should be made by an informed consumer. Sometimes a savvy, well-traveled WOW is better off handling her own holiday arrangements.

Many of those reduced fares, discounted hotel rooms, and less expensive dinners start at age fifty. If you've passed that milestone and haven't as yet responded to your AARP invitation, you might want to mail that form in now! At many hotels across America, simply flashing an AARP card will entitle you to substantial savings.

Crossing in Style

If you're willing to sail on standby, you can even get a bargain on the *QE II*. Flexibility and a spur-of-the-moment spirit of adventure may enable you to take advantage of the dramatically reduced fares offered in the ship's Standby to Europe program. The price includes the five-day crossing aboard the completely refurbished queen of the sea and a one-way airline ticket home from London to any one of eighty-two U.S. cities. You'll receive confirmation of your reservation a month ahead of the crossing date. If you are traveling with a companion, the cost can be as low as $1,500 per person; single cabins are available for $100 more.

WHEN TO MISS THE BOAT

You don't want to cruise as a single WOW aboard a ship of foolish women on the lookout for a husband. Hey, I loved *Now, Voyager*, too, but Bette Davis didn't meet Paul Henreid on the Carnival Line.

Research any ship that you're considering as if you were inspecting the *Titanic* for possible leaks. If possible, go down to the dock and watch the male passengers as they board. Check out their average age and demeanor. As a rule of thumb, the more madras Bermuda shorts and T-shirts you spot on the gangplank, the less promising your prospective shipmates will be.

On most cruises—both tacky and upscale—there are so many older, unescorted women that the ships actually employ retired men as dance hosts. The job description? They must be presentable as well as able to walk, talk, and waltz the wallflowers around the ballroom. None of the lines hires Wonderful Older Women to dance with extra men. There are never any of them on board.

How to Choose an Appropriate Travel Partner

Two can travel cheaper than one, but traveling in pairs is like a mini marriage. European hotel rooms are very tiny. Make sure your fellow traveler's grooming and sleeping habits won't have you ending up your vacation in a foreign prison! Husbands are usually a safe bet. Be wary of going off with a new man in your life. Waking up in Rome and deciding you can't room with a man who never puts the cap back on the toothpaste tube or snores loud enough to be heard in Naples is no way to spend a holiday.

If there's no man in your life, or even if there is, another WOW

Seven Ways to Save When You Sail Away

1. Travel on cruise lines that include any airfare in the cost of the cruise or that offer a substantial savings on plane tickets.

2. Look for two-for-one deals. Two can sail for the price of one or the second passenger goes for 50 to 70 percent off.

3. Book a less expensive inside cabin. You're only there when you're sleeping, and you may be able to upgrade to a classier cabin, complete with porthole, if the ship doesn't have a full complement of passengers upon embarkation.

4. Seek out specials. Some lines provide a free night at a hotel before boarding and/or upon return to shore.

5. Reserve and pay for your accommodations at least six months in advance. Many ships offer up to a 50 percent discount for early birds.

6. Or do the exactly the opposite: Book a cruise a week before the scheduled sail date. On many lines the still passengerless cabins will be cheaper by half.

7. Best bargain of all: Do what I did and sail for free! Lecture or teach aboard ship. Turn your hobby, career, or area of expertise into a free passage. What a deal for a WOW. Theme cruises are in need of experts in various areas from art to zoology. Bridge instructors, financial planners, and psychics can cruise for free, paying only the port charges, along with golf pros, swing dancers, and travel mavens. And as more and more Americans are sailing off into the sunset, the cruise lines' entertainment directors need more and more onboard talent.

Maybe, based on my previous experience lecturing aboard the *QE II*, I can take *Foxy Forever* across the Atlantic!

makes a great roommate. Unless she's a Category A friend and you've traveled together before, don't fly off to another continent on your maiden journey. Test the arrangement with a weekend jaunt. See if you can live with her on or near your own turf before venturing abroad; it makes a quick exit easier.

Even though it's tough to find tours where you won't have to pay double for the privilege of sleeping alone, on some trips paying a higher price for privacy can save your sanity. You can go where you want when you want; eat breakfast in bed while reading the local paper without conversation; take as long as you like in the bathroom; and if on a tour, chat with whomever catches your fancy.

Except for eating dinner at a table for one, I rather like traveling alone. And I've learned to challenge any restaurant maître d' who seats me in Siberia. Many Wonderful Older Women have come face-to-face with restaurant discrimination and been stuck with their backs to the rest of the room, staring at a kitchen door. Over the last decade most restaurants have wised up, treating women going solo as well as they'd treat a man dining alone. And long before that, while traveling in London, I felt as if the hosts and waiters showed no sexual preference.

When a Bargain Is a Bad Deal

While we all want to find a tiny jewel of a hotel or inn that is clean, comfortable, and cheap, here's a tip: Unless someone whose opinion you value has stayed there, don't make reservations at any place that promotes itself as "quaint" or "charming." It probably has a bathroom down the hall and no hot water. (Incidentally, that same caveat about "quaint" and "charming" holds true when those words are used to describe real estate.)

Once at a bargain hotel in Paris there was no elevator, my room was on the second floor, and the only bathtub was on the fourth. When I complained, the concierge said, "But madame, your room has a bidet."

While we shouldn't conspire to make travel abroad seem just like being at home, Americans are big on creature comforts: showers, electrical outlets, room service, lots of fluffy towels, telephones, and television. Quaint ain't. And for some of us that's okay.

However, I'm such an anal-retentive pain in the butt that my friend Vesna Ostertag Beck, both worldly and a world traveler, advised me, "Stay out of Egypt!"

"You mean I may have to die without seeing the pyramids?"

Vesna shrugged. "Maybe you can cruise the Nile and never get off the boat."

The Sidewalks of New York

I seek my own slow pace in any traveling companion. My niece, Susan, another snail, and I spend four to five days in Carnegie Hill every August when it's hot, sticky, and everyone in his right mind and his psychiatrist has escaped from Manhattan. We go for those very reasons: Hotel rooms are readily available and inexpensive, the streets are relatively empty, and theater tickets are on two-fers; and minus the crowds, you can see all the paintings at the Metropolitan Museum of Art and hang out for as long as you like.

Carnegie Hill is a gem of a New York neighborhood where tourists seldom stray or stay, thus missing out on one of the best bites of the Big Apple. Bounded on the west by Fifth Avenue and Central Park, on the east by Third Avenue, on the south by Eighty-sixth Street, and on the north by Ninety-eight Street, it contains some of New York's priciest real estate. The Hill is known as Museum Row.

The limestone-and-brick mansion on Fifth Avenue and Ninety-first Street, modeled on an English Georgian home and built by Andrew Carnegie at the turn of the twentieth century, now houses the Cooper-Hewitt Museum, a New York wing of the Smithsonian. The Guggenheim (Frank Lloyd Wright's concrete egg, filled with modern art), the National Academy of Design (America's fashion parade presented as cultural exhibits), and the Jewish Museum (Judaica treasures and traditions) are all within a few blocks' walk.

But best of all is the Hotel Wales and Quik Book's bargain rates.

The Wales . . . *there's a small hotel* . . . is the best bed-and-breakfast in Manhattan. Located at 1295 Madison Avenue and opened in 1901, the building, featuring an eclectic facade with stone balconies, round-arched windows, and decorated escutcheons, is an intriguing architectural hodge-podge. Check-in takes place in a small, elegantly refurbished reception area. However, the real lobby is the grand salon on the second floor; it is filled with potted plants and has geraniums on the sills of lace-curtained windows, and its Victorian settees and walls are covered with paintings by some of the finest turn-of-the-century children's artists. An oak side-board provides a great breakfast, including peach preserves and freshly baked breads. Every afternoon, tea and cookies are offered, together with a concert at five. On Sundays a string quartet plays to a full house. Think Jane Austen.

Most of the rooms at the Wales are small; in August, so is the cost. If you use Quik Book (1-800-789-9887) to reserve, you can save up to 60 percent off regular rates. During our last stay we upgraded to a suite, which was filled with charm and less than a standard room in season. And it's nice to visit Carnegie Hill in the style it deserves.

See the U.S.A.

But not on a tour bus filled with senior citizen complainers. There is nothing wrong with senior citizens. By the time you're reading this, I will have officially, joined their ranks. I just don't want to go on a long trip with people who have chosen to travel in an age-segregated vehicle. And I don't much like buses, either.

Attending an Elder Hostel program with my peers is one thing; crossing Colorado in a tour bus is quite another.

As for the complaining, I recall working the lecture circuit of the condos in Broward County while promoting *Contestant.* From that ex-perience I've decided that when too many older people live for long pe-riods of time in communities populated only with their peers, kvetching is raised to an art form. Imagine what it might be like in the close quarters of a tour bus before you take that trip to Branston!

Going It Alone

Travel with a purpose. If your destination is a spot like Williamsburg, Virginia, where you can devour a slice of history or a trek through the theaters of London or a long weekend at a bed-and-breakfast on New England's coast, don't have any qualms about going alone. All you need is a purpose, a plan, and some common sense.

A purpose provides you with the opportunity to create a travel agenda that will be so intriguing and so tailored to your interests that you'll be glad you're on your own. You'll be doing exactly what you want, where you want, and when you want. And your fellow tourists will share your enthusiasm for the area, or they wouldn't be there. So if you do want to strike up a conversation, the opportunity and the common bond will be available.

When a WOW travels alone, planning is paramount. Make sure all your arrangements are airtight. Follow a well-thought-out itinerary. Do you have an up-to-date map of the area? Will a van from your hotel meet you at the airport? Is a continental breakfast included in the daily rate? Will you dine before or after the theater? Does the B&B have an afternoon tea? The latter could be important in timing your afternoon's sightseeing. Tea can be both a source of comfort and a social hour where you can spend some time chatting with the other guests.

Safety features in a hotel or inn should be considered. Rooms located off an inside hallway are safer than those with an entrance from the outside. Hotels with a card-key system—usually in large cities—are more secure, and no matter where you're staying, good locks are essential. So is a telephone in your room. And is there someone on staff, even if it's a small inn, who is always available? When you're driving to your destination, make sure the parking area is close to the building and brightly lighted.

Get going! You'll probably have the time of your life all by yourself. After all, a WOW is good company.

Adventure Ahead

Exotic excitement and thrill-a-minute trips aren't only for the young and daring. A WOW can live just as dangerously. Well, some of us can. Count me out of traveling to any destination that doesn't have indoor plumbing. It started the summer I turned twelve and spent the month of August at camp with five other Girl Scouts sharing a buggy tent and one ghastly outhouse. And it still holds true. Not too long ago someone told me that my idea of the great outdoors was "the space between the hotel lobby and the taxi."

If you've always wanted to climb the Himalayas, canoe over the rapids at the Delaware Water Gap, balloon over Borneo, bike through Brussels, or drive a jeep while on safari in Kenya, there's a travel agency that will tailor the trip to your taste for adventure and whisk you off to anywhere in the world. An incipient WOW, Gloria Stuart, president of Atlas Travel, Fort Lauderdale, says, "The globe's your playpen."

As for me, once again this August I'm going to explore the Metropolitan Museum of Art and Central Park. Maybe this year I'll visit the zoo.

The Second Time Around

Many of us Wonderful Older Women are now grandparents who diapered the last of our own children over a quarter of a century ago. We thought we were finished with parenting. Now we're either welcoming back our post-college-age sons and daughters while they "find themselves"—though it might be better if what they found was a job—or powdering babies' buns as we find ourselves raising our kids' kids.

Hi, Mom, I'm Home . . . Again!

After her daughter had married and her son had been graduated from college and accepted a position in Atlanta, Doris Holland celebrated by adopting two dogs. "This will be the first time in twenty-five years that I'll be totally on my own! The dogs will keep me company." Yet she also fretted over missing the "children." She need not have worried! Her kids kept coming home for years, sometimes bringing along a husband or a fiancée, but always bringing along their cats and dogs. Now that JP is married and living nearby in his own home, it's unlikely that he'll be returning. However, Jennifer is divorced and, after a long hiatus studying in Greece, will be back again this summer. "Just between sessions."

Naturally nurturing and full of energy, Doris thrives on this revolving-door policy. Other Wonderful Older Women—often living in smaller quarters—wish their adult children would feather their own nests.

The Family of the Future

Statistics indicate that almost 10 million Americans over the age of forty-five now share nontraditional living arrangements. According to a 1992 report from the U.S. Census Bureau, almost 60 percent of these households are made up of some combination of what we refer to as extended families, such as the Hollands'. Another 6 percent reflects grandparents as caregivers in the absence of the children's parents.

Is this the trend of the future? It certainly looks that way. There is no question that in the next census the numbers will be much higher and the problems will be much more complex.

Where are the parents? Why can't they raise their own children? If the grandparent is the primary caregiver, with complete financial, medical, moral, and social responsibility for her/his grandchildren, what are her/his legal rights regarding those kids?

A few years ago Renee Woodworth, director of AARP's Grandparents Information Center, spoke at a House of Representatives' Older Americans Forum about the problems confronting grandparents and how AARP has been trying to help. "We know that more than three million children are living in households headed by a grandmother or grandfather—and a million of those are being *brought up* by a grandparent."

These caregiving grandparents—and today those numbers are even higher—often are caught in a legal morass, discovering that although the kids have become their responsibility, they may have no right to register them for school, obtain financial aid, sign for necessary medical treatment, or take the kids out of state.

Most of the parents of these children are among the missing—strung out on drugs, in jail, sick with AIDS, or virtually vanished. But those parents who are a quasi-presence can present an even worse problem. If the child lives with his grandparents but they and the parent(s) are not getting along, the child will pick up on the family feud, further impairing the three-way relationship. And should the grandparents be taken to court and be removed from the grandkids' lives, the situation can become really frightening. Sometimes the parent whisks the child out of state, and the grandparent never sees her/his grandchild again.

On the December 12, 1998, *Today Show*, Dr. Arthur Kornhaber from the Foundation for Grandparenting said about these kids, "If the grandparent leaves their lives, they not only resent the parents, but fear they will dump them, too."

Dr. Kornhaber stressed the importance of a new federal law protecting the visitation rights of grandparents.

Talking to Wonderful Older Women who are taking care of their grandchildren, I learned about the Grandparents' Rights' Advocacy Group (GRAM) founded by Pat Slorah in Tarpon Springs, Florida, in 1999. Started as a support group, GRAM morphed into a political action group that changed Florida's legislation regarding grandparents' rights. Another active group, founded by Miriam Horn, is GRO—Grandparents Reaching Out—on Long Island.

Must reading material includes Dr. Lillian Carson's *The Essential Grandparent*, geared toward America's fastest-growing segment of the population—those of us raising children for *The Second Time Around*. And I learned that General Colin Powell is the national spokesperson for grandparents. He's a good man to have on the side of a WOW grandmother.

A Good Man Nowadays Is Hard to Find

Or like the old joke—and a much more difficult search: A hard man nowadays is good to find.

The over-fifty single scene: Is it really the lowest level of Dante's Inferno? Abandon hope, all ye who enter here?

I have now visited church socials, single sailing clubs, and fifty-plus dances from New York City to Palm Beach and from there to the Washington area. Yes, many of these events were truly *hell*—the Jesuits can start rethinking eternal damnation—but some of them were quite a lot of fun when I remembered to follow my own ABC + PEAK steps. When I practiced what I preach, I had a great time, though I never met the man of my dreams or even my nightmares. (In case you've forgotten the WOW foxy forever formula—ABC + PEAK—return to Chapter 3 immediately!)

By the Sea

The sailing clubs gave over-fifty sports a ship and a common interest to share. These were far better and more fun than most of the "socials" that I attended where everyone knew that what you were angling for was a date.

At the Fort Lauderdale Single Sailing Club, a crew, usually three guys and three gals, would be assigned to a captain, and if all went well, soon all aboard would be steering into the eye of the wind. A grand adventure. I never met a mate, but lots of Wonderful Older Women have. And if you love the ocean, don't get seasick, and are willing to wear shorts, sailing off into the sunset could land you a date with destiny.

Dancing in the Dark

A woman in my condo in Florida divorced an attractive, amusing, affluent man because he wouldn't go dancing five nights a week. Then to take her husband's place, I presume, she installed a wooden platform and mirrored the den so she could properly practice her tap dancing routine.

"Oh, he'd go to a ballroom one or two nights," she told me during our exercise class in the pool, "but dancing is my passion. Now I can go six nights a week. And I've found a new partner. Why don't you come with us one night?" Since I thought her husband appeared to be a pretty cool guy, I was wondering just what kind of a high this gal got from twirling around the floor. I was about to find out.

My neighbor met me in the lobby. She wore a black-and-white prom dress complete with crinolines and color-coordinated shoes, bag, and earrings. I wore beige silk pants and a matching man-tailored shirt. It was a good bet that I would be the most dressed down Cinderella at the ball.

Explaining to the prom queen that between dances I would be doing research for *Foxy Forever*'s chapters on the single scene for Wonderful Older Women, I brought along a pad and pen.

These notes were taken while I sat among the other wallflowers at Mr. Dance, a "ballroom" located in a strip mall:

A multicolored ball dangling from the ceiling spins, casting rainbow hues around the huge room. Most of the ladies are sixty-something, and most of them are dressed like either demure bridesmaids or glittery hookers. Most of the far more casually dressed gentlemen are seventy-something; however, there's a good sprinkling of extremely agile octogenarians. As they slide, swing, dip, and twirl, dancing into death, I realize how inadequate my fox-trot is. And my only-used-at-weddings waltz won't cut a rug with this bunch. I'm prepared to remain a wallflower. Hell, this is research. I don't have to be Scarlett O'Hara. Like a war correspondent, I only want to observe, not become part of the action.

But before I can sip on my ice water, which is the ballroom's drink of choice, a prospective partner appears.

I dance nine times with nine different partners. No one asks me for an encore performance. I'm not up to Mr. Dance's usual standards. One guy—who looks like a B movie gigolo—offers to teach me. "Private classes. Very reasonable." I have potential, he says, if no rhythm. He can have me dancing the bossa nova in three lessons or less. He bows and hands me a greasy business card.

The men explain their dancing styles as they attempt to get me to follow their lead. "I'm a street dancer," says one. "Self-taught. Learned my routines in the forties on the sidewalks of New York." He jerks a thumb at a couple who glide by like Fred and Ginger. "I'm not one of them. They're too studied. Suffering from dance studio lessons!" Actually, I think they look great. And everyone is having, you should pardon the pun, a ball.

I don't think Prince Charming is ever in residence at Mr. Dance's. And forty-somethings who never touched each other while learning how to dance and who wouldn't know a peabody from a cakewalk will probably never want to swing at Mr. Dance's ballroom. When these dancers gracefully whirling around me segue into that great ballroom in the sky, there will be no one to lindy hop in their place. I smile when the ninth man returns to ask me for a second time around the floor.

Wow, was I ever wrong! A year or two later the swing dancing craze swept the country. Tacky ballrooms spruced up as Generation Xers jammed their floors, dancing cheek-to-cheek with their grandparents who stayed a step ahead of them. I'm reconsidering those lessons!

The Beat Goes On

In my relentless north-to-south-to-mid-Atlantic pursuit of a good man, I may not have ended up married, engaged, or going steady, but I did have several super sails, a few good dinners, and one wickedly wonderful waltz to remember. Yes, at a ballroom.

Whenever I revealed that I was doing research for a book, I found myself surrounded by bookworms and sundry literary types. It's a great opening line; you have my permission to use it. A caveat: Most of my "admirers" just wanted to know how I'd found an agent.

I've come to the conclusion that the best way to find a man is not to look. Yet like the goddess Diana, I enjoy the hunt. It's catching one that spoils the fun.

The truth is I want a date for dinner, not someone to hover over me while I apply my makeup. Or click the remote every millisecond. Or talk while I'm reading. Or read while I'm talking. I'm not in the market for a full-time husband, and based on the appallingly poor results of my man-hunt, that's a damn good thing.

Even when only searching (or researching) for a part-time partner who might in a crisis be able to change a battery or jump-start a car, *A Good Man Nowadays Is Hard to Find!*

So Where Are Those Wonderful Older Men? Can a WOW Meet a WOM?

My search garnered so much information, if nary a warm body, that it led to a south Florida production company's decision to shoot a pilot for a television show—with me as host—geared toward older women and called appropriately enough, WOW. Since I was sick of talk shows about people eager to date their cousin's cows, and since there were no talk shows skewed toward topics that would interest the WOW population, I felt the timing was right. The program's concept, much like the foxy forever formula, would chart a course for a happy, healthy, and exciting journey to old age. PBS in Miami evidenced some strong interest. I rounded up a panel of experts. All were single, sister Wonderful Older Women whom I knew and respected. And "A Good Man Nowadays Is Hard to Find" became the first topic for the pilot's taping.

Now, as they say on television news and talk shows, in terms of full disclosure, WOW never made it on the air, and I still haven't found a man—good, bad, or indifferent. However, the advice offered during that show's interviews, the honest exchanges among the panelists, and the startling changes that took place in the lives of my WOW guests are not only well worth sharing but are totally amazing.

Four Wonderful Older Women shared the spotlight with me. Martha Gross, the sixty-something, longtime society editor for the *Fort Lauderdale Sun-Sentinel,* had published four romance novels, for and about people over fifty. She served as poet laureate for Hollywood, Florida, had hosted a radio show, was a frequent public speaker, and three years before, at the age of sixty, had become a part-time circus aerialist. I'd asked Martha because she epitomized Wonderful Older Women and because she'd recently brought four dates to a wedding. While I'd felt that was a tad greedy, I found it almost as fascinating as Martha's swinging through the air with the greatest of ease!

Dr. Anne Mulder, a former college president and a nationally known educator, speaker, and writer, served as professor of higher education for Nova Southeastern University. Anne, in her early sixties, believed that most of the older men she'd encountered in south Florida dated only miniskirts. However, Anne was in the throes of an international long-distance love affair with a man whom she'd met in Greece while on vacation—a man twenty years younger!

Sue Florio had worked with me in the admissions department at the Art Institute of Fort Lauderdale. She was also my beach buddy. We had spent long hours lounging in the sunshine, unknowingly increasing our wrinkles along with deepening our tans, while swapping stories of our past and present dates. More often it was the lack of same. The conclusion reached during those seaside conversations: Our future romantic possibilities in sunny Florida looked pretty gloomy.

My fourth guest, Joan Mazza, held a master's degree in counseling and was a licensed mental health counselor who led workshops in dream appreciation and journal writing. As the author of *How to Meet Your Mate Through the Personal Ads*, Joan appeared as an "expert" who would advise the WOW panel on how best to solve the south Florida shortage of good men.

It's really a shame PBS turned thumbs down on WOW in favor of a sports program. Never have five women been more candid on camera. The audience, mostly Wonderful Older Women who were sipping tea at Ireland's Inn, Fort Lauderdale, while the pilot was being shot, loved it. So did the director and the production staff, but as with a good man, we couldn't find a television channel that had a head of programming brave enough to "skew old."

The Romance-Wanted Ads—AKA "Personals" and "Dial a Date"

Martha's four dates but no romance; Anne's younger man who lived on another continent, though eventually love conquered geography; Sue's saga of her forty-one dates from hell; my sad songs of looking for love in all the wrong places and then wondering why I met all the wrong men; and Joan's upbeat advice on how a personal ad can bring romance entertained and informed.

"Meeting people through the personal ads offers you a way to be really clear about what you want in a relationship," Joan Mazza told the panel. "My best advice: Be your *real* self. Don't lie about your age, looks, or circumstances. The truth is bound to come out later and undermine what might have been a good relationship. Why would you want someone who has fallen in love with his fantasy instead of you?"

Sue and I decided to listen to Joan and try the personal ads. I'd gone

that route in New York with no success, but for Sue they were virgin
territory. Hey, we weren't doing too well on our own. How bad could
they be?

Joan also strongly suggested that a WOW should be the one who
places the ad. The responses would provide an opportunity to winnow
out the losers. But based on my previous New York experience with these
ads and priding myself on being discerning enough to weed out nuts,
phonies, and the improvised, I opted to answer.

Can a WOW Wearing Bifocals Read Her Way to Love?

The following are actual ads that I didn't answer. Not a word is changed.
You couldn't make this stuff up.

SWPM—LATE 50s

Educated, handsome, millionaire producer, beach front home,
yacht, international travel, looking for a ten—great in a bikini—
18–30.

MAN OF GOD

Christian man, 53, 5'11", 180 lbs, seeks three things from God:
a ministry, a mate, and a million dollars. Seeking Christian female, 40s–mid 50s, petite/medium build, who desires a Christian
lifestyle.

AGE NO BARRIER

Lovable senior, early 70s, 5'9", 217 lbs, in top form, seeks person
20–45, for long-term friendship/relationship.

SLOOP DU JOUR

Height 72", width proportioned to length of 56', world-traveled,
smashing when all dressed up, needs woman's touch. Oops! Sa-
crebleu! Almost forgot. French Capitaine comes with her. Hope
you like!

Here's one I *did* answer, even though by no stretch of the imagination could my 5'3" be considered tall.

HELP! HELP!

Rescue a DWCM, recently alone, tall, intelligent, Ivy League, monogamous, relaxed gentleman seeks SWCF, 50+, tall, attractive, intelligent, monogamous significant other with a touch of class.

I met him at a local restaurant overlooking the Intercoastal. Tall, very tall. A Yale graduate. Full of himself and gin. And, since retiring, glued to his regular seat at the bar, which faced away from the water. Fifteen minutes after saying hello, I faked a headache and walked home . . . alone. Single blessedness had never felt so good.

Over the next two weeks I answered three more ads. They were all "nice" guys—a kiss-of-death description—and therefore not for me. One of them, an ex-fighter pilot who had written a novel, enrolled in my How to Get Published class and has remained a friend. Another looked like a younger Ronald Reagan, was a native New Yorker, and quite chatty. I thought he might have possibilities, but he, too, seemed to be drinking his way through retirement. The third, a former IBM executive, seemed to have it all: good-looking, a great dancer, and a fun—if powerful—personality. We met three times, a record for me. On our last date my personality crashed head-on with his. I never heard from him again.

However, Sue did!

The Greater Fort Lauderdale area, despite the Chamber of Commerce's best effort to promote it as a thriving city, remains a small town. How many men over fifty-five could there be running around loose and placing ads? Sue, unbeknownst to me, had also met and discarded both Mr. Ivy League and Mr. Ronald Reagan look-alike. Comparing notes on our dates while sitting in the sand and staring at the ocean, she shared with me that the latter had spent most of the evening talking about me, said he'd loved my hair. Good thing the ersatz Mr. Reagan was already history in Sue's date book.

Mr. IBM was a different story. He had captured her heart, and a little over a year later, Sue Florio married Jim Gwinn, and I went to their wedding. Still without a date.

Joan Mazza moved right along to electronic dating. She met a guy through an Internet personal ad. He flew from West Virginia to Fort Lauderdale to rendezvous with her; however, after meeting him, Joan decided "his e-mails were more exciting than he was."

On her fiftieth birthday Joan hosted a celebration for twenty of her friends. I felt delighted to be among the Wonderful Older Women who shared in Joan's "coming of age" party. At the candle-lighting ceremony Joan said, "You each are a light in my life!" What a memorable ritual! The bonding was sincere, and the love around that table was palpable. Not to mention the acquired knowledge and the wisdom of those women who gathered to honor Joan's passage.

A short time later *Dreaming Your Real Self: A Personal Approach to Dream Interpretation* hit the bookstores' shelves and has been flying off them ever since. Joan's officially a WOW, and so is her book.

Dr. Anne Mulder recently caught up with me for tea at the Four Seasons Hotel in Washington. Her speaking engagements and educational seminars keep her busier than ever, flying around the country and abroad. She's a loving mother, a doting grandmother, and a working WOW who is now married to her much younger Greek Adonis. I'm not kidding—that's his name.

Martha Gross is flying high, too. Successful and happy. And her romance novels are delighting her readers. What else would you expect from a WOW who had four single men seated at her table at a wedding reception?

As for me, I'm still a SWDF: *looking for a long-term—but part-time—relationship with a literary, witty, wise older man who possesses style and class.*

I'll Take Romance

When you find him, what do you do with him? What does he do for you? And together can you do "it"?

At fifty, the author Colette declared that she would never make love again after catching a peek at herself in the mirror while doing "it." Poor Colette should have turned out the lights and done "it" by Braille. *N'est-ce pas?* One would think that the sexy creator of *Gigi* would have acquired far more wisdom and imagination.

Romance can conquer age, though the anticipation of doing "it" can still make a WOW feel like a teenager. What's wrong with that? Older women perform better sexually than older men. Just ask us. And atrophied vaginas are no deterrent. An over-the-counter lubricant works miracles. If we're lucky, occasionally our lovers perform the miracles.

However, a WOW's best sex and biggest miracle might be courtesy of Viagra.

So will your sex life still sizzle in your sixties? Did it ever? If it did and if you have the right partner or can find one, your accumulated sexual expertise as well as your foxy forever attitude should keep those orgasms coming—through your sixties, seventies, eighties, and, if you haven't killed him by then, your nineties!

An Old Wife's Tale

An eighty-two-year-old WOW who wishes to remain anonymous told me that she and her husband of almost sixty years set a date for sex once a week. Erotic literature, candles, wine, scented satin sheets, Josephine Baker's records on the "Victrola," and a vibrator are on hand. The couple established this sex playtime thirty years ago when their youngest child left home. Smiling, the attractive WOW said, "Sometimes Saturday night is so good that he has his hand under my skirt as we're heading out to church the next morning."

"And this was before Viagra?" I asked.

"Lord, yes. He just tried that for the first time last month. All those Bob Dole ads, don't you know? Jim respects Dole; they both served in World War II. Looks like we'll be adding at least one more night each week."

"What's your secret for great sex?"

"No secret. He's good in bed." She laughed, crinkling her bright blue eyes. "And with all the practice, I'm pretty good at 'it' myself."

SEX AND THE SINGLE WOW

A baby boomer turns fifty every seven to eight seconds, and divorce or sometimes death boomerangs many a WOW back into the single scene. Being a celibate young single is tough enough; sex can throw a single WOW in a quandary.

Since a woman's chance of remarrying after forty continues to be much lower than her chance of being hijacked by a terrorist, an over-fifty WOW's chance of finding a desirable man for doing "it" probably ranks lower than a shot at going to the moon.

I remain a romantic—I cry at Hallmark commercials—but I'm also a realist. The good guys, as we've established, are in short supply. And though not wanting to be married should be an asset, possibly making a prospective beau feel less threatened, often it isn't.

Doris Holland's ongoing belief that "a twenty-hour-a-week relation-ship is perfect" continues to greatly exceed my ideal relationship time frame. Much as I would welcome a significant other—God, how I hate that term—in my life, I prefer a good murder mystery or the *Times* cross-word puzzle with my tea and toast. On the other hand, being all dressed up with somewhere to go is always better if you have someone to escort you there.

I have long suffered from the *Casablanca* curse syndrome. I need to keep reminding myselt that Rick Blaine, in his impeccably tailored white dinner jacket and running that gin mill in the Casablanca of the early forties, is, after all, a fictional character.

It could be that *I'll Walk Alone* as I have for almost twenty-five years. And since my remaining single seems to be more by choice than chance, *It's Okay with Me!*

Many of the older men who are alive and out there looking for a "relationship" are also looking forward to being married. They actually *want* to have breakfast with the woman/wife of their dreams. But these men may not be the stuff that a WOW's dreams are made of.

"For God's sake, this guy I met playing tennis proposed on the third date!" one WOW complained. "I really liked him, but with that much mileage on him, I felt he needed a test drive. I told him we had to sleep together before I'd consider marrying him!"

"What did he say?" I asked.

"Nothing." She shrugged. "Last April he married my doubles partner. They were divorced two months later."

Sexual Behavior

"The best sex occurs in our fifties, sixties, and seventies," according to Pat Love, a relationship therapist. Appearing on the January 29, 1999, *Today Show*, Love told Katie Couric that the ads for Cadillacs and Centrum Silver feature sexy seniors because a lot of seniors are sexy. Her advice: Deal with who you are as you mature. Accept yourself. A lot of people say that confidence is the sexiest thing of all. Don't look at the past. Start again. After fifty, men and women become more of a match in their sexual goals. Pat Love warns that lifestyle—drinking, smoking, being overweight—catches up with those of us over fifty and advises that one of the ways to a healthy sex life is to have open discussions with our doctors.

SEX AND STATISTICS

Most older Americans remain sexually active into their eighties. Some for much longer. The National Council on Aging report published in late 1998 indicated that 74 percent of the men and 70 percent of the women over sixty found their sex lives more emotionally satisfying as seniors than they had when they were in their forties. And 39 percent said they were happy with the amount of sex they were having—even when it was none. Another 40 percent said they wanted to make love more often.

This, of course, is great news for Wonderful Older Women in stable relationships. But statistics regarding the rise in sexually transmitted diseases, from the American Social Health Association, are scary. The panel concluded that there were 15.3 million new cases reported in 1996—up 3 million from a decade earlier.

A WOW is not immune. *AIDS has no age limit.* Just before I left Florida, a senior citizen and AIDS activist made the rounds of local television shows to warn other older women who were returning to the world of romance that they'd better be practicing safe sex. This attractive widow hadn't been promiscuous, only trusting. And foolish. She'd reentered the dating game. Her new partner had lied, and she had believed him. Then she was diagnosed as HIV positive and bravely decided to tell her story to the world—hoping to prevent other Wonderful Older Women from making the same foolish mistake in the name of love.

Her plight and her courage reached me. Sitting alone in my living room, I watched that woman's despair and listened to her message. A message for all Wonderful Older Women—one that might save our lives.

I made an appointment with my doctor. It was time for my yearly checkup anyway. I liked my doctor; she was another WOW. I decided to have my first and—so far—only HIV test. Though I had no real reason to suspect I might have a positive result, I suddenly felt irrationally worried, guilty, and embarrassed. Like Hester must have felt when they stuck that scarlet A on her chest. Like the Catholic schoolgirl I'd once been.

The Irish talk a lot. They love a lively discussion and will venture an opinion on almost anything. Just not about sex. My father would ask me to leave the room—even after I'd been married—if he thought someone was about to tell an off-color joke.

On the way to the doctor's office I realized that I hadn't been so nervous since my sixteenth summer when I'd indulged in some heavy petting and had to figure out how to slip that major fall from grace in among my other less interesting sins during confession. But as a teenager I didn't have to worry about birth control or condoms: I never would have gone all the way. What if I became pregnant? How could I have confessed that to either God or my father?

Now here I was, almost a goddamn senior citizen, sweating an AIDS test. What a revolting development the sexual revolution had turned out to be!

THE TEST

That sunny afternoon when I reached the doctor's office, I was so crazed that I should have been meeting with a shrink instead of an internist. My doctor seemed somewhat surprised that I'd never been tested before and asked me a few questions. My incoherent answers, knee-jerk reactions, and insistence on CIA-style cover, including complete confidentiality and using an alias, which necessitated setting up a second file, sending the blood sample to a private lab, and not filing an insurance claim, didn't seem to daunt the good doctor. However, after taking my blood pressure, she did suggest I might try to calm down. She then left the room, saying that she'd be right back. I flew into a full panic attack when a good-looking young man wearing scrubs and carrying a needle appeared in her stead.

"Who are you?!" I shrieked.

He smiled. Confidently. "I'm the nurse. I'm going to take your blood."

That's what he thinks, I thought. I wanted to kill Dr. Batista. How could she have turned me over to this callow youth for such an important procedure?

After spending several shaky minutes explaining to the nurse that my file for this test had to be classified as top secret and kept separate from my real identity, he calmly assured me that he understood—completely.

Then he marked my new folder Ms. Doe and promised to call me as soon as the results came back from the lab.

I let him draw my blood.

THE RESULTS

A few days later the nurse called with the results of my HIV test. Negative. The irrational and inexplicable guilt was gone instantaneously. I apologized for being such a nut case. He said he understood and wished me well—and sounded as if he meant it. I could pick up the hard copy of the test results when convenient, and there would be no report in my medical file. Ms. Doe had vanished along with my fear.

Fortunately, most Wonderful Older Women are handling this simple test far better than I. If we remain single and sexually active, we should be tested regularly and always use what one WOW referred to as "condom sense."

The Romantic Aftermath

Years ago the book *Six Months with an Older Woman* not only entertained me as a bittersweet love story but gave me hope that someday I would get to spend six months with a younger man. And as karma would have it, I did. Well, actually five months and three and a half weeks.

Toward the end of my hunt for one good man, I dragged my fellow writer and sister WOW Gloria Rothstein along with me to a singles party in Boca Raton. Fifty or more mostly over-forty folks crammed the living areas and patio of an upscale home not far from the beach. The gal who ran these events had cajoled her friends into donating their home. Other parties were held monthly at country clubs and included dancing. Sometimes she'd host a lecture or theme event. That night it was strictly a social. You paid your twenty-five dollars and received a modest buffet, a glass or two of wine, and a chance to mix. And, with any luck, make a match. Based on the large turnout, Gloria and I figured our hostess had made a quick profit.

As these things go, this party proved to be above average. It provided an opportunity to talk to some well-dressed professional men, several of whom surprised me by crossing the room to start a conversation.

My younger guy was one of them. What he strode across was the patio, where I'd gone to catch my breath and a bit of fresh, if humid, air. With thick white hair, blue-gray eyes, a Robert Taylor profile, and a flat, firm stomach, he almost took away the breath I'd just recovered. I gulped, then grinned, realizing that I'd resigned myself to never feeling this way again.

When his call came a few days later, his dinner invitation had my adrenaline and hormones pumping like a teenager's. We went to a restaurant on the ocean and afterward took a walk on the beach, then settled into chairs on the patio and talked until two in the morning. He was into New Age. I was closing in on what some might define as old age, and though he didn't know it, I'd turned eighteen the year he was born. Our first date was Saturday night of Memorial Day weekend. He invited me to go to the movies with him on Monday.

I'd arranged to meet yet another "ad" man on Sunday. Driving to the country club in Del Ray, all I could think about was the night before. My luncheon companion didn't have a chance—even if he hadn't been an old bore who probably had someone else draft his personal ad. He lived in a gated community, so quiet and well tended that it reminded me of a cemetery.

Back home by three, heart aflutter, I dialed my Saturday night date's number. It had been years since my last romance. I didn't want to wait until Monday.

He took me to action movies; I read him the chapters from my murder mystery in progress.

About a month into our relationship I said, "You do know that I'm a lot older than you."

He told me that a woman from the singles party who had once been interested in him mentioned that possibility. "But not old enough to be my mother?" he asked. I just laughed.

I broke up with him after my test results. Since the news had been good, I still don't know exactly why. He'd been tested less than a year before we met and had only one sexual encounter since then. That's not good enough; both partners should be tested at the start of any sexual relationship. He assured me that I was the only woman currently in his life, yet I couldn't get beyond how foolish and frightened I felt.

If romance ever reappears in my life, I'll think with my head before following my heart.

Love and Marriage

Paul Newman and Joanne Woodward. Diane Sawyer and Mike Nichols. Sophia Loren and Carlo Ponti. Bob and Elizabeth Dole. Elizabeth and Philip. Al and Tipper Gore. All the Bushes. All high profile. All long married. All still happy?

A lot of Wonderful Older Women have stayed married to their first or second husbands for decades. Are they still happy in long-term wedlock? And what's it like when you took him for better or worse and now, due to downsizing or retirement, you're stuck at home alone with him underfoot twenty-four hours a day? How do you cope? Can couples be *too* close?

Many other Wonderful Older Women—the widowed and the divorced, even some longtime singles—are contemplating a trip down the aisle, some after years of living on their own. What does a late-in-life merger do to our psyches, our privacy, our families, our friends, and our finances?

Is having a warm body (who probably snores) in bed with you and an almost-guaranteed-for-life Saturday night date worth the price? A surprising number of us are saying yes.

And with multiple marriages, just which husband do we get to spend eternity with? Is heaven a ménage à trois? I think I'd like to solo on my cloud; however, that may be because some people who are so sure they're going to heaven are such bores. Widowers tend to sing the praises of their late wives, sometimes too often, to their second wives. What will be a remarried widower's seat preference on his heavenly cloud assignment?

I took a close look at several of these women, ranging from recent brides to those about to celebrate their fortieth or fiftieth anniversary. All of them shared their love stories with honesty and humor.

Hanging In

The children and I plan to celebrate Joe's seventieth birthday in Ireland during the millennium.

—Bernice Crudden

I asked Bernie, "Why did your marriage last?"

"That reminds me of the early seventies when we used to sit around with cheap wine asking, 'What is life?' " she said with a laugh. "The wine is more expensive now, but I still have no real answers."

"Still, something made it work," I persisted.

"What worked for us might be all wrong for other couples. We gave ourselves a lot of space; we're both very independent people. But we also have a strong sense of family, including extended, and we can both handle compromise, which is important to our relationship because our interests are so diverse." I knew that to be true. Bernie and Joe have canceled out each other's vote in every presidential election since they've been married. "And we both rely heavily on the other's integrity."

We were conducting this interview long distance. Bernie and Joe live in Dallas. But as always when speaking to Bernie, it seemed as if there was neither space nor time separating us.

So many of my old friends' marriages have ended in divorce, but the Cruddens' relationship has thrived. And so have their four children. At their daughter Colleen's wedding, one of the groomsmen said, "You guys are the perfect parents. With Joe playing his guitar, the family sing-alongs, and the kids in their homemade Halloween costumes, your home movies look like reruns of *Leave It to Beaver*."

Bernie and Joe met in 1949 and had a fun-filled, carefree fifties courtship. She remembers it fondly. "Today, no one, no matter what age, ever seems to be that young and carefree. When Joe was a junior at Drexel, I was chosen fraternity sweetheart, a big event in my life. We married on Valentine's Day in 1952 because we were very much in love and because it was so romantic—and that date would, I thought, help him remember our anniversary. But after forty-seven years, he still forgets."

As Joe made inroads in his successful engineering and sales career, the young couple moved often. And the first thing Bernie would do after settling in their new home was join the local theater group. While raising the kids, she turned her hobby into a career, appearing in regional theater, print and TV ads, national television shows, and currently "doing lots of retirement home commercials!" Her daughters followed in her footsteps, and by the time they landed in Dallas, all three were actresses and models.

As a couple in "retirement," they're busier than ever. Joe left his job, but he still does international consulting. "Maybe his being away so much all those years helped the marriage," Bernie said.

Several years ago she started a second career as a wedding coordinator, turning her well-honed hostess skills into a paying profession, and has done very well. And they travel around the world, often visiting friends Joe made when he was abroad on business.

"Our kids met people of every nationality—from Europe, the Far East, and Australia—by helping us entertain Joe's clients whenever they came to Dallas. This gave the children a broad perspective on people and life that is reflected today in their own lifestyles." Bernie said that she and Joe are proud of and close to their four children and their "eight beautiful grandkids, all of whom have Irish names!"

But she felt there was a lot of luck involved in making her family life so happy. "Tom Brokaw has called the generation before mine the Greatest Generation. I call ours the Luckiest Generation. We were too young for World War II, just missed the Korean War, and then were too old or too married with children for Vietnam. The economy was booming as Joe started his career, and his financial success made our lives easier. Our sons were too young for Vietnam and too old for the Gulf War. And, hey, there's even some Social Security money still there for us!"

Finally, Bernie cited compatible genes as possible factors in the success of her forty-seven-year marriage. "I'm a big believer in genes! I think that Joe and I were both born with a 'happy' gene and a 'commitment' gene. We're both very positive about most things. We've always looked for the silver lining, and we believe in hanging in. Of course, we love each other deeply, and speaking for myself, I've never met anyone else that I'd give him up for."

As I hung up the phone, I felt much better about Wonderful Older Women in long-term marriages.

Speak for Yourself, Karen!

World War II ended in mid-August 1945; Karen Cahill Bartholomew arrived exactly nine months later, making her one of the first of the baby boomers. Decades later, Karen, along with thousands of other boomers, had to reinvent herself after her divorce. During her long marriage to a doctor—they'd been college sweethearts—she was a stay-at-home mom and then enjoyed some success as an actress in Washington and New York. Single again and over forty, Karen knew she had to find a less capricious and more permanent career. She went back to school, obtained her master's degree, and became a psychiatric social worker. No doubt her stage skills helped her when she interacted with her patients.

When her two children left home, Karen, who enjoyed the company of men, decided that she might reprise the dating game. Would she ever consider getting married again? Well, maybe, if she found the right guy. The search was on!

Knowing that Washington, D.C., could be barren territory for a middle-age manhunt, Karen turned to the personal ads. We compared our worst experiences. Karen won hands down. I drew the nerds. She attracted the nuts.

"So I met this guy for coffee," Karen said. "He showed up looking

like an unmade bed on parade, and a full four inches shorter than the
five feet nine inches that he'd claimed to be. He opened the conversation
by saying he would only date a woman who earned over fifty thousand
dollars a year. Then, smiling gleefully, he boasted that he had several file
cabinets with over two hundred files on the women he'd met through the
personal ads. As you can imagine, this made me really nervous. I bolted.
Never even said good-bye! I couldn't wait to get home and change my
phone number. Thank God he didn't have my last name!"

This experience severely soured her on the "personals."

Then her best friend and my niece, Susan Kavanagh, came across an
ad that might be a perfect match for Karen. "Just an Irishman with a tie."
The woman of his dreams would be "attractive, 5'7", with dark hair and
blue eyes." The writer of that personal ad had described Karen.

"I'm not responding to one more ad!" Karen said. So Susan answered
it for her, and when Michael called, Karen liked what she heard and
made plans to meet him. After their second date, Susan made a suggestion: "There are too many women out there. If you like him, make your
move." Karen invited Michael to the Kennedy Center.

He told me, "I walked into the lobby that night and saw this beautiful
woman dressed like a dream and offering me a glass of wine. I was a
goner." They were serious enough by the fourth date for Karen to accompany him to his law firm's convention. They moved in together soon after
that and were married a year later.

They have five children between them. One of them is always coming
home, being driven to college, graduating, or setting up housekeeping in
another city. Karen and Michael seem to thrive on their travels and on
their mutual love: Its glow lights up their faces.

Recently, and just in time for my *Foxy Forever* interview, they moved
into the same Washington, D.C., co-op where Susan and I have apart-
ments. That move will turn our traditional Christmas night journey to
dinner at their house into a short ride in the elevator.

I've been in love with Diane for over thirty years!
—Dave Dufour on his wedding day,
October 7, 1989

In 1957, *The Stars Fell on Alabama* played on jukeboxes and radios across Massachusetts while two teenagers in a Boston suburb rode the school bus, stealing glances, but never speaking to each other. Although Dave Dufour had been a "super jock," he traveled with a "fast" crowd who defied the rules. Diane Dowling Dufour now admits, "I would never have started a conversation. Though certainly intrigued, I was afraid of him!"

Dave says, "She was the prettiest girl in the school and from the swanky side of town; I knew I didn't stand a chance."

By 1958, Diane was a senior and Dave had graduated, married, and fathered his first son. Their paths wouldn't cross again for more than twenty years. Each was married and divorced twice. Dave had three children; Diane had two. Neither one was in the market for a relationship when, on a golfing vacation in Fort Lauderdale in 1980, Dave called Diane and invited her to dinner. "I was so surprised to hear from him!" Diane said. Dave had been following her life via the grapevine since high school. He'd wrangled her phone number from a mutual acquaintance in Boston. They met and talked about old times, though they had none in common, and then returned to the lives they'd been living.

Diane next ran into Dave in 1985. Fort Lauderdale is a small city. She was involved with someone else. So was he, but he was on a holiday alone. They spent a pleasant hour together catching up. His next phone call came in 1986. By then Diane was living with that someone else.

In January 1989, Dave showed up once again. In addition to chasing after golf balls he chased after Diane. In romance as in life, timing is everything. Both were at liberty. Dave didn't have to rush back to Boston, and Diane, who had always been attracted to him, thought he looked better than ever. And all their friends, including me, said they made a striking couple. For health reasons, Dave had stopped smoking years before, and as fate would have it, Diane had just gone to a hypnotist to quit, too.

A week into daily dating, they were ready to get married! Diane wanted to wait until her youngest daughter finished college. They decided to hold the wedding in Key West and invite family and friends to join them in a weekend of parties. But they had a hell of a time finding a special day that they could call their own, a date on which to celebrate their anniversary in all the years to come. A date that neither had been married or divorced on. A date that none of their children had been born on. A date that no one dear to either of them had died on. Third marriages can present some challenges.

Their day turned out to be October 7, 1989. Key West hotels and rooming houses were filled with Diane and Dave's wedding guests. From Dirty Harry's prenuptial eve blast to the beautiful and spiritual poolside ceremony and the great reception that followed, it was a wedding weekend to remember.

And after more than a decade of marriage, Diane and Dave—the self-described odd couple—are still celebrating life and love, even on days that belong to someone else.

The World Series Wedding Reception

They had seemed an unlikely match: Vesna Ostertag, a cosmopolitan woman born in Europe, a Ph.D. and an international educator whose interests were arty and intellectual, and Bill Beck, a guy from Kansas City whose entire life and career had centered around baseball. She'd traveled the world, spoke several languages, and managed to be fascinating and funny in all of them. He was the traveling secretary for the Florida Marlins. They met in Fort Lauderdale. Rosalie Bernstein, happily married herself and an intrepid, unrelenting matchmaker, had introduced them one still sunny evening after work in the summer of '94. I watched them fall in love.

As different as they were, Vesna and Bill had many similar qualities. Both were warm and caring; both had generous hearts and loving souls; both were loyal to their families and friends, and true to their spiritual values. In many ways they were the perfect match.

Vesna threw great parties, mixing multicultural college professors with third basemen. Her elegant condo overlooking the Atlantic was as close to a salon as south Florida would ever entertain. She was a happy woman, and she made those around her happy, too. Especially Bill.

In November '97, two months after the Marlins won the World Series, Vesna and Bill flew to Hawaii and were married on the beach. That January they hosted a reception at the Tower Club in Fort Lauderdale. Diane Dowling Dufour acted as wedding coordinator, turning the already beautiful room into a fairy-tale setting: The theme was seashells and baseball, and the international jet set got to dance with the world champion players.

And as wedding favors, all the guests took home sterling silver seashells holding vials of sand taken from the beach where the bride and groom had been married—and photographs of themselves taken during the reception while holding the World Series winners' trophy!

The Largest and Oldest Wedding Party in the Bridal Book of Romance

When Barbara Rasche was widowed, she never suspected that a new romance with her husband's old friend would sweep her off her feet. She and Richie had been married a lot of years when he had a fatal heart attack while playing softball. Like most long marriages it had had some rocky patches, but they'd hung in. Barbara had branched out into a successful career as a salesperson on Seventh Avenue in New York's famed wholesale garment district. Tall, very attractive, and always smartly dressed, at fifty-something Barbara could have passed for one of her showroom's models.

Many of the mourners who attended Richie's funeral at Saint Bartholomew's in Manhattan had attended Barbara and Richie's wedding in that same church thirty years earlier.

Still feeling lost and lonely, Barbara returned to work. She had a daughter in college and a son planning to be married. I remember our flying together to Michigan—and joking about being each other's date—for the wedding of Barbara Crowley-Giorgio's oldest son. That weekend in a motel filled with old friends, Barbara and I were roommates. We reminisced and we laughed a lot, but we cried, too. And during one late-night pajama party, we promised each other that if either of us ever got married again, the other would be a bridesmaid at the wedding.

When Barbara returned to New York, she received a call from Jack Kelly, who had grown up on the same block as her late husband and was himself a widower. They began what I called a telephone courtship. When they finally went out on a date, the romance really moved along. Jack told Barbara that he'd admired her from afar for decades.

Shortly after her son's wedding, just as she and Richie had planned, Barbara sold her house and moved to Stuart, Florida. To no one's surprise, Jack sold his house on Long Island and followed her. About a year later Barbara and Jack were planning their own wedding. And remembering our pajama party, Barbara invited five of her oldest (literally) and dearest friends to be members of the wedding. And Jack asked his brothers and his old friends. Two of them, conveniently, were married to two of Barbara's bridesmaids. Then Barbara asked her daughter and Jack's daughter. Including the bride and groom, that added up to a wedding party of *sixteen*!

During the rehearsal at Saint Mary's Episcopal Church in Jensen Beach, I asked the priest if this was the oldest—I felt certain we were the craziest—wedding party he'd ever been involved with. He responded, "Not the oldest but definitely the largest!"

Our old crowd—most had attended Barbara's first wedding—traveled from Texas and California and Michigan and New York to celebrate Barbara and Jack's marriage—and to admire the over-fifty bridesmaids who were wearing sea-foam green taffeta gowns with shoes dyed to match. The groomsmen were dashing, too, in their tuxes, as we all marched into the reception to unbridled applause and a standing ovation. The guests were old enough to voice how happy they were to be together at a wedding, not a funeral, and young enough to twist the night away, dancing until dawn.

We all stayed at the hotel, located right on the beach, for a weekend of parties. There seems to be a pattern in older brides' wedding celebra-

tions: They last for several days, celebrating life, love, and longtime friendships.

I'm happy to report that love and marriage are still in full bloom among
Wonderful Older Women.

Autumn Leaves

What lies behind us and what lies before us are
small matters compared to what lies within us.
  —Ralph Waldo Emerson

A WOW is strong, resilient, optimistic, and realistic. In almost any situation that might confound a twenty-something, a WOW has been there and done that. Yet most of us are not jaded. Or bored. Or apprehensive. We're enjoying where we're at, but we're ready for the scene to change. Prepared to take our places onstage for Act 3, certain that it will be our championship season.

From Mary Malloy, calmly confronting the final battle that her husband of forty years faced with Alzheimer's who made the tough decisions, together with their five children, while working to keep the bills paid on time; to Agnes Kelly, who lost her beloved son but remained a source of strength for his four siblings and her husband; to Karen Bartholomew, the oldest Ph.D. candidate at Smith College, while coping with a new career, new husband, and their combined young adult children—a WOW inspires.

A WOW may have money woes—far too many do—but somehow manages. A WOW may have health problems but somehow accepts and deals with them. A WOW may be raising two, three, or more grandchildren but somehow manages and copes. Wonderful Older Women never cease to amaze.

In the Indian summer of our lives we display our colors proudly: the golds, russets, and burnt siennas of autumn. We remain rich in spirit, ripe for adventure, and ready to plan for a winter of content. We impart wit and wisdom on mundane trips to the supermarket as well as at glamorous dinner parties. We bring a touch of elegance to a world sorely in need of style and substance.

And when we reign as the first young-old generation, by being foxy forever we will change the way America looks at aging.

WOW!

About the Author

Noreen Wald has worked as an essayist, editor, seminar developer, lecturer, and writing instructor and has previously published three books, *Contestant*, *Ghostwriter*, and *Death Comes for the Critic*. She currently resides in Washington, D.C.